Lecture Notes in Statistics 151

Hamid, Stefan Israelsson, Kristi Kuljus, Johan Lindbäck and Habte Tewoldeberhan for their constructive criticisms of the manuscript as well as for pointing out several errors. The lecture notes were re-written taking their comments into account during the second half 1999. We are also grateful to the referees of Springer for careful reading and numerous constructive suggestions on how to clearify bits and pieces as well as language improvement. Needless to say, the authors are responsible for any remaining errors. Tom Britton gratefully acknowledges support from the Swedish Natural Science Research Council.

Håkan Andersson, Stockholm *February, 2000*
Tom Britton, Uppsala

Contents

Part I

STOCHASTIC MODELLING

In the first part of these lecture notes, we present stochastic models for the spread of an infectious disease in some given population. We stress that the models aim at describing the spread of viral or bacterial infections with a person-to-person transmission mechanism. Diseases that belong to this category are, for example, childhood diseases (measles, chickenpox, mumps, rubella, ...), STD's (sexually transmitted diseases) and less severe diseases such as influenza and the common cold. Diseases excluded from these models are, for example, host-vector and parasitic infections although they have some features in common. Modifications of epidemic models can also be used in applications in the social sciences, modelling for example the spread of knowledge or rumours (see e.g. Daley and Kendall, 1965, and Maki and Thompson, 1973). In this context being susceptible corresponds to being an ignorant (not having some specific information) and infectious corresponds to being a spreader (spreading the information to other individuals). One possible rumour model is where the spreader continues to spread the rumour forever which corresponds to the SI model (e.g. Exercise 2.3).

Two main features make the modelling of infectious diseases different from other types of disease. The first and perhaps most important reason is that strong dependencies are naturally present: whether or not an individual becomes infected depends strongly on the status of other individuals in its vicinity. In Section 1.2 we shall see how this complicates the stochastic analysis, even for a very small group of individuals. For non-transmittable diseases this is usually not the case. Occurences of such diseases are usually modelled using survival analysis, in which hazard functions, describing the age-dependent risk for an individual to fall ill, are specified; proportional hazards (Cox, 1972) is an important example. These hazards may be specific to each individual and even contain a random parameter which may be correlated between related individuals; as in frailty models (e.g. Hougaard, 1995). Even then the disease-times for different individuals are defined to be independent given the hazard functions, contrary to the case for infectious diseases. A thorough analysis of such models and their statistical analysis, including many examples, is given in Andersen *et al.* (1993).

The second feature, which affects the statistical analysis, is that most often the epidemic process is only partly observed. For example it is rarely known by whom an infected individual was infected, nor the time at which the individual was infected and during what period she was infectious (here and in the sequel we denote individuals by 'she'). Problems related to this property are treated in Part II of the lecture notes.

In the introductory chapter we present the simplest stochastic model, discuss advantages and disadvantages of stochastic models as opposed to deterministic models and give a brief overview of the history of epidemic models and give some general references on epidemic modelling. In Chapter 2 we define what we call 'The standard SIR epidemic model' (SIR epidemic for short), which serves as the canonical model in the text. The abbreviation SIR is short for 'susceptible', 'infectious' and 'removed'. SIR models assume that individuals are at first susceptible, if they get infected they remain infectious for some time, after which they recover and become immune. An individual is said to be removed if she has recovered and is immune or dies, and plays no further role in the epidemic. A construction of the SIR model is given in Chapter 2, and exact results concerning the final size (i.e. the total number infected by the disease) and 'the total area under the trajectory of infectives' are derived. In Chapter 3 the Coupling Method is presented, a method which enables the SIR epidemic model to be approximated by a branching process during its initial stage, assuming a large population. First, the main idea of coupling is given, and then it is applied to the SIR epidemic model. In Chapter 4 the important threshold limit theorem, concerning the final size of the SIR epidemic in a large population, is stated and proved. In Chapter 5 we are concerned with approximations of the entire epidemic process and not only its final size. This relies on diffusion theory for the special case when the epidemic model is Markovian.

Chapters 6 and 7 extend the standard SIR epidemic to the case where the population is not completely homogeneous. Chapter 6 is devoted to so-called multitype models, where individuals are of different 'types' and these types differ, for example in terms of susceptibility. In Chapter 6 we also model the spread of disease when the community is built up of households, assuming different transmission rates between individuals depending on whether they belong to the same household or not. In Chapter 7 we characterise an epidemic model in terms of random graphs. This technique is introduced to model heterogeneities caused by e.g. social structures or geographic location. The last chapter of Part I, Chapter 8, concerns models for endemic diseases, i.e. diseases which are present in the population over a long period of time. The models of this chapter are different in that new susceptible individuals have to enter the population for endemicity to occur. This can be achieved by assuming that old individuals die and new (susceptible) individuals are born into the population, i.e. a dynamic population, or that individuals become susceptible after recovery rather than immune. The latter type of model is, for obvious reasons, called an SIS model.

1 Introduction

1.1 Stochastic versus deterministic models

These lecture notes focus on stochastic models and their statistical analysis. Deterministic epidemic models have perhaps received more attention in the literature (see also Section 1.4 about the history of epidemic models). For example, the monograph by Anderson and May (1991), probably the most cited reference in the recent literature on epidemic models, treats almost exclusively deterministic models.

The main advantage of deterministic models lies in their simpler (but not necessarily simple!) analysis. For a stochastic epidemic model to be mathematically manageable it has to be quite simple, and thus not entirely realistic. Deterministic models can be more complex, yet still possible to analyse, at least when numerical solutions are adequate.

Several reasons suggest that stochastic models are to be preferred when their analysis is possible. First, the most natural way to describe the spread of disease is stochastic; one defines the *probability* of disease transmission between two individuals, rather than stating certainly whether or not transmission will occur. Deterministic models describe the spread under the assumption of mass action, relying on the law of large numbers. In fact, an important part in stochastic modelling lies in showing what deterministic model the stochastic model converges to, when the community size becomes large. Secondly, there are phenomena which are genuinely stochastic and do not satisfy a law of large numbers. For example, in a large community, many models will lead either to a minor outbreak infecting only few individuals, or else to a major outbreak infecting a more or less deterministic proportion of the community (see Section 1.3 below). To calculate the probability of the two events is only possible in a stochastic setting. Further, when considering extinction of endemic diseases (see Chapter 8), this can only be analysed with stochastic models, since extinction occurs when the epidemic process deviates from the expected level. A third important advantage concerns estimation. Knowledge about uncertainty in estimates requires a stochastic model, and an estimate is not of much use without some knowledge of its uncertainty.

To conclude, stochastic models are to be preferred when their analysis is possible; otherwise deterministic models should be used. Deterministic models can also serve as introductory models when studying new phenomena. We see no conflict between the two and believe that both types of models play an important role in better understanding the mechanisms of disease spread. In these lecture notes we focus on stochastic models, for deterministic models we refer the reader to Anderson and May (1991), and Bailey (1975) – who also treats stochastic models.

1.2 A simple epidemic model: The Reed-Frost model

Before describing some general characteristics of the models to be studied, we present the simplest possible epidemic model for the spread of an infectious disease, say the common cold, in a small group of individuals. The model is called the Reed-Frost model named after its founders (see Section 1.4 on the history of Epidemic modelling) and is a so-called chain-binomial model (also treated in Section 10.2). The model is an SIR epidemic model which means that individuals are at first *susceptible* to the disease. If an individual becomes infected, she will first be infectious, and called an *infective*, for some time and then recover and become immune, a state called *removed*. An individual is said to be infected if she is either infectious or removed, i.e. no longer susceptible.

The model is usually specified using discrete time dynamics. In the discrete time scenario it is natural to think of the infectious period as being short and preceded by a longer latent period. Then new infections will occur in generations, these generations being separated by the latent period as the discrete time unit. The event probabilities in a given generation depend only on the state of the epidemic in the previous generation (i.e. a Markov model), and these events are specified by certain binomial probabilities. If we let X_j and Y_j denote the number of susceptibles and infectives respectively at time (or generation) j, the chain-binomial Reed-Frost model has conditional probabilities

$$\begin{aligned}&\mathbf{P}(Y_{j+1} = y_{j+1}|X_0 = x_0, Y_0 = y_0, \dots, X_j = x_j, Y_j = y_j)\\&= \mathbf{P}(Y_{j+1} = y_{j+1}|X_j = x_j, Y_j = y_j)\\&= \binom{x_j}{y_{j+1}} (1 - q^{y_j})^{y_{j+1}} (q^{y_j})^{x_j - y_{j+1}},\end{aligned}$$

and $X_{j+1} = X_j - Y_{j+1}$. This means that a given susceptible of generation j remains susceptible in the next generation if she escapes infection from all infectives of generation j; these events are independent each occurring with probability q. Further, different susceptibles in a given generation become infected independently of one another and infectious individuals are removed in the next generation. Given the initial state $X_0 = n$ and $Y_0 = m$ the probability of the complete chain $y_1, \dots, y_k, y_{k+1} = 0$ is obtained by conditioning sequentially and using the Markov property of the chain. If we let $x_{j+1} = x_j - y_{j+1}$ we have

$$\begin{aligned}&\mathbf{P}(Y_1 = y_1, \dots, Y_k = y_k, Y_{k+1} = 0|X_0 = n, Y_0 = m)\\&= \mathbf{P}(Y_1 = y_1|X_0 = n, Y_0 = m) \times \cdots \times \mathbf{P}(Y_{k+1} = 0|X_k = x_k, Y_k = y_k)\\&= \binom{n}{y_1} (1 - q^m)^{y_1} (q^m)^{n-y_1} \times \cdots \times \binom{x_k}{0} (1 - q^{y_k})^0 (q^{y_k})^{x_k}.\end{aligned}$$

From a mathematical point of view, the spread of the disease does not have to occur in generations. The necessary assumption is that each individual who becomes infected has 'infectious contact' with any other given individual (meaning that the individual becomes infected if she is still susceptible) with probability $p = 1 - q$, and all such contacts occur independently. Of course, the notion of generation becomes less meaningful, unless there is a long latency period prior to the infectious period. Still the formula can be used when computing the total number of infected individuals $Z = \sum_{j\geq 1} Y_j$, as we shall see (note that the initially infectives m are excluded). The quantity Z is also known as the final size of the epidemic.

To compute $\mathbf{P}(Z = z|X_0 = n, Y_0 = m)$ we simply sum the probabilities of all chains for which $|y| = \sum_{j\geq 1} y_j = z$. From the defining equations it is seen that $Y_j = 0$ implies that $Y_{j+1} = 0$. This means that new infections may only occur whenever some individuals are infectious, which implies that the length of a chain cannot be longer than the total number infected, making the number of possible chains finite. The probability function for the final number infected is hence

$$\mathbf{P}(Z = z|X_0 = n, Y_0 = m) = \sum_{y:|y|=z} \mathbf{P}(Y_1 = y_1, \dots, Y_k = y_k, Y_{k-1} = 0|X_0 = n, Y_0 = m).$$

Below we calculate the probability function explicitly for Z, the final number infected among those initially susceptible, when $Y_0 = m = 1$ and $X_0 = n = 1$, 2, and 3. Since $m = 1$ in all cases we omit it in the conditioning notation. We start with $n = 1$:

$$\begin{aligned}\mathbf{P}(Z = 0|X_0 = 1) &= \mathbf{P}(Y_1 = 0|X_0 = 1) = q,\\ \mathbf{P}(Z = 1|X_0 = 1) &= \mathbf{P}(Y_1 = 1, Y_2 = 0|X_0 = 1) = p.\end{aligned}$$

For $n = 2$ we have

$$\begin{aligned}\mathbf{P}(Z = 0|X_0 = 2) &= \mathbf{P}(Y_1 = 0|X_0 = 2) = q^2,\\ \mathbf{P}(Z = 1|X_0 = 2) &= \mathbf{P}(Y_1 = 1, Y_2 = 0|X_0 = 2) = \binom{2}{1} pq \times q,\\ \mathbf{P}(Z = 2|X_0 = 2) &= \mathbf{P}(Y_1 = 2, Y_2 = 0|X_0 = 2) + \mathbf{P}(Y_1 = 1, Y_2 = 1, Y_3 = 0|X_0 = 2)\\ &= p^2 + \binom{2}{1} pq \times p.\end{aligned}$$

For $n = 3$ we compute only the first three probabilities, the final probability may be derived from the complement.

$$\begin{aligned}\mathbf{P}(Z = 0|X_0 = 3) &= \mathbf{P}(Y_1 = 0|X_0 = 3) = q^3,\\ \mathbf{P}(Z = 1|X_0 = 3) &= \mathbf{P}(Y_1 = 1, Y_2 = 0|X_0 = 3) = \binom{3}{1} pq^2 \times q^2,\\ \mathbf{P}(Z = 2|X_0 = 3) &= \mathbf{P}(Y_1 = 2, Y_2 = 0|X_0 = 3) + \mathbf{P}(Y_1 = 1, Y_2 = 1, Y_3 = 0|X_0 = 3)\\ &= \binom{3}{2} p^2 q \times q^2 + \binom{3}{1} pq^2 \times \binom{2}{1} pq \times q.\end{aligned}$$

Needless to say, these probabilities become very complicated to compute even for moderate sized groups (n larger than 10 say). The Reed-Frost model is a special case of the standard SIR epidemic model presented in Chapter 2, in which the length of the infectious period is deterministic (implying that contacts between pairs of individuals occur independently). As for the model of Chapter 2, we implicitly assume that the population is homogeneous and that individuals mix homogeneously. In Section 2.4 we derive the final size probabilities in a more coherent way for the more general model.

1.3 Stochastic epidemics in large communities

The previous section illustrates the need for approximation methods when considering large communities. In fact, the recursive formulas for the final size presented in Section 2.4 are numerically unstable and cannot be applied to obtain numerical solutions when the number of susceptibles n exceeds 50-100.

The main insight from such large population approximations is the threshold limit theorem (Chapter 4). Loosely speaking, this theorem states that, as $n \to \infty$ one of two possible scenarios can occur: either a) only few individuals will ever become infected, or else b) a more or less deterministic positive *proportion* of the susceptibles, with some Gaussian noise of smaller order, will have been infected by the end of the epidemic. The latter scenario is referred to as a large or *major* outbreak. Much work has been carried out to state versions of this theorem for more and more general models, and in particular to derive the probabilities of each of the two scenarios as well as finding the deterministic proportion infected in case of a large outbreak. Another important task is to find out for which parameter values the asymptotic probability of a major outbreak is 0. The parameter R_0, called the basic reproduction number, plays a crucial role in this context. The parameter R_0, a function of the model, is the average number of new infections caused by a 'typical' infective during the early stages of the epidemic. The threshold limit theorem states that a major outbreak in a large population is possible if and only if $R_0 > 1$. From a statistical perspective only major outbreaks are considered since minor outbreaks would rarely be observed at all. Questions of interest are then to derive parameter estimates, including their uncertainty, having observed the number of infected. The main motivation for such estimation lies in the control of disease spread. If for example a vaccine is available, a question of practical relevance is to estimate what proportion of the susceptible population it is necessary to vaccinate, in order to avoid future outbreaks, a state known as 'herd immunity'. This type of question is considered in Chapter 12.

Sometimes not only the final state of the epidemic is of interest, but rather the entire epidemic process. It is then possible to approximate the epidemic process using diffusion theory (see Chapter 5). This is, for example, the case in the statistical setting where data is collected continuously from an ongoing epidemic, a topic treated in Chapter 9.

1.4 History of epidemic modelling

This section will give only a short selected presentation of some early mathematical models for the spread of infectious diseases. We have no intention of covering all important events in the development of this subject. For a more detailed historical overview we refer the reader to the books by Bailey (1975) and Anderson and May (1991).

One of the earliest studies of the non-linearity of an epidemic model was contained in a paper by Hamer (1906). Hamer postulated that the probability of a new infection in the next discrete time-step was proportional to the product of the number of susceptibles and the number of infectives. Ross (1908) translated this 'mass action principle' to the continuous time setting. The first complete mathematical *model* for the spread of an infectious disease which received attention in the literature was a deterministic model of Kermack and McKendrick (1927). This model, known as the deterministic general epidemic, is now presented (note that the parametrization is different from the models treated later in the text). Let $x(t)$, $y(t)$ and $z(t)$ respectively denote the number of susceptibles, infectives and removed (=recovered and immune, or dead) individuals. The population is considered to be of fixed size n (i.e. $x(t) + y(t) + z(t) = n$ for all t). The model is then defined by the following set of differential equations

$$\begin{aligned} x'(t) &= -\lambda x(t)y(t) \\ y'(t) &= \lambda x(t)y(t) - \gamma y(t) \\ z'(t) &= \gamma y(t), \end{aligned} \tag{1.1}$$

with initial state $(x(0), y(0), z(0)) = (x_0, y_0, 0)$. In Figure 1.1 we show how (x, y, z) varies over time for $\lambda = 1.9$ and $\gamma = 1$ where the bottom region corresponds to $x(t)$, the middle region to $y(t)$ and the top region to $z(t)$ (which is empty at $t = 0$ since $z(0) = 0$). Note that their sum remains constant over time since $x(t)+y(t)+z(t) = n$. The factor $\lambda x(t)y(t)$ in (1.1) is the crucial non-linear term, indicating that infections occur at high rate only when there are many susceptibles *and* infectives. From the first two equations it follows that $dx/dz = -\theta x$, where $\theta = \lambda/\gamma$. So $x(t) = x_0 e^{-\theta z(t)}$ and hence $y(t) = n - z(t) - x(t) = n - z(t) - x_0 e^{-\theta z(t)}$. Kermack and McKendrick (1927) showed that y is decreasing unless $y_0(\lambda x_0 - \gamma) > 0$ or equivalently $x_0 > 1/\theta$. In this latter case there will be a growing epidemic. This observation is known as the threshold result, i.e. that completely different behaviour will occur depending on whether x_0 exceeds $1/\theta$ or not. Another important observation was that $z(t) \to z_\infty < n$ as $t \to \infty$, where z_∞ is the solution of $z = n - x_0 e^{-\theta z}$. This leads to the very important property that not everyone becomes infected!

The first stochastic model was proposed by McKendrick (1926). This model, a

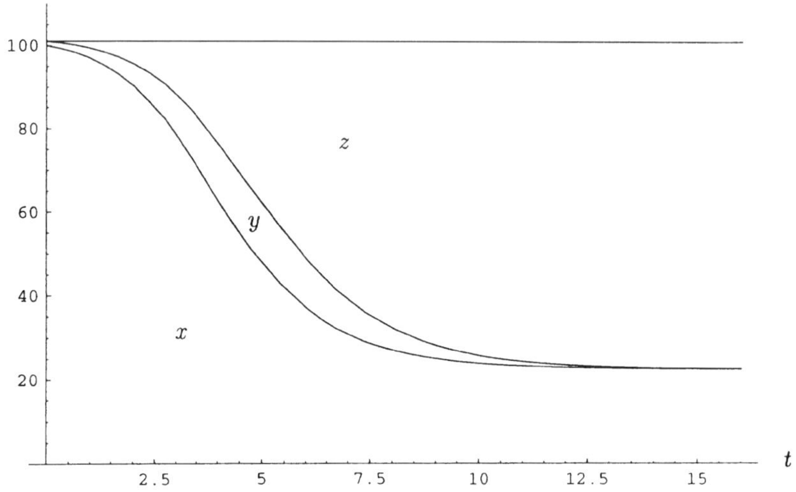

Figure 1.1: Plot of $(x(t), y(t), z(t))$ defined by (1.1) with $\lambda = 1.9$, $\gamma = 1$, $x_0 = 100$ and $y_0 = 1$. For each t, $x(t)$ corresponds to the lower segment, $y(t)$ to the mid-segment and $z(t)$ to the top-segment. (N.B. $x(t) + y(t) + z(t) = 101$ for all t.)

stochastic continuous-time version of the deterministic model of Kermack and McKendrick (1927), did not receive much attention. A model which attracted more attention at the time, even though it was never published, was the chain-binomial model of Reed and Frost (presented in Section 1.2) put forward in a series of lectures in 1928.

It was not until the late 1940's, when Bartlett (1949) studied the stochastic version of the Kermack-McKendrick model, that stochastic continuous-time epidemic models began to be analysed more extensively. Since then, the effort put into modelling infectious diseases has more or less exploded. In the rest of the lecture notes a selection of these methods will be presented.

The list of references covering epidemic models and their analysis can of course be made long. Here we only mention a few central texts. The first pioneering monograph was written by Bailey in 1957 but has since then been reprinted in a second edition (Bailey, 1975). This book covers both stochastic and deterministic models as well as statistical inference with numerous applications to real data. Becker (1989) is mainly concerned with statistical analysis of infectious diseases. Gabriel *et al.* (1990) is a collection of papers, on stochastic modelling and some statistical inference, that were written for a workshop on stochastic epidemic modelling in Luminy, France. The book by Anderson and May (1991) mentioned previously is probably the book which has received the most attention, together with Bailey (1975). Anderson and

May (1991) model the spread of disease for several different situations and give many practical applications. The book is also concerned with estimation; however, both modelling and inference are deterministic. A thematic semester at Isaac Newton Institute, Cambridge, resulted in three collections of papers (Mollison, 1995, Isham and Medley, 1996, and Grenfell and Dobson, 1996), covering topics in stochastic modelling and statistical analysis of epidemics (i.e. its propagation in a community), human infectious diseases (i.e. the infection process inside the body), and animal diseases, respectively. Very recently, two new monographs have been published. The first one is written by Daley and Gani (1999) who have a long experience in stochastic modelling of the spread of disease. This book focuses on stochastic modelling but contains also statistical inference and deterministic modelling, as well as several historical remarks. Diekmann and Heesterbeek (200?), finally, are concerned with mathematical epidemiology of infectious diseases and also apply their methods to real data.

Exercises

1.1. Compute $\mathbf{P}(Z = 0|X_0 = 10, Y_0 = 1)$, $\mathbf{P}(Z = 1|X_0 = 10, Y_0 = 1)$, $\mathbf{P}(Z = 2|X_0 = 10, Y_0 = 1)$ and $\mathbf{P}(Z = 3|X_0 = 10, Y_0 = 1)$ for the Reed-Frost model. (Hint: Compute the probability for each epidemic chain giving $Z = k$ separately and then add these probabilities.)

1.2. Show that $y(t) \to 0$ as $t \to \infty$ for the model of Kermack and McKendrick given by the differential equations (1.1).

1.3. Consider again the Kermack-McKendrick model and assume $x_0 > 1/\theta$. Using the formula $y(t) = n - z(t) - x_0 e^{-\theta z(t)}$, show that the maximum number of infectives occurs exactly at the time t when $x(t) = 1/\theta$.

2 The standard SIR epidemic model

In this chapter we present a simple model for the spread of an infectious disease. Several simplifying assumptions are made. In particular, the population is assumed to be closed, homogeneous and homogeneously mixing. Also, the effects of latent periods, change in behaviour, time varying infectivity and temporary or partial immunity are not taken into account. In later chapters we shall indicate ways of handling some of these complicating features of a real-life epidemic.

2.1 Definition of the model

We assume that initially there are m infectious individuals (that have just become infected) and n susceptible individuals. The infectious periods of different infectives are independent and identically distributed according to some random variable I, having an arbitrary but specified distribution. During her infectious period an infective makes contacts with a given individual at the time points of a time homogeneous Poisson process with intensity λ/n. If a contacted individual is still susceptible, then she becomes infectious and is immediately able to infect other individuals. An individual is considered 'removed' once her infectious period has terminated, and is then immune to new infections, playing no further part in the epidemic spread. The epidemic ceases as soon as there are no more infectious individuals present in the population. All Poisson processes are assumed to be independent of each other; they are also independent of the infectious periods.

We call this model the *standard SIR epidemic model*, the letters S, I, R standing for the terms 'susceptible', 'infectious' and 'removed', respectively. Following Ball (1995), we denote the process by $E_{n,m}(\lambda, I)$. Also denote the mean and the variance of the infectious period I by ι and σ^2, respectively. The rate of contacting a given individual is set to λ/n in order to keep the rate at which a given infective makes contact with other (initially susceptible) individuals constant ($= \lambda$), independently of the population size. The special case where the infectious period has an exponential distribution will be discussed in some detail further on.

The basic reproduction number and the final epidemic size, already encountered in the Introduction, are two extremely important epidemiological quantities. The final size of the epidemic, Z, is simply defined as the number of initially susceptible individuals that ultimately become infected. Thus Z is a finite random variable taking values between 0 and n. In Section 2.4 we shall derive a linear system of equations for the distribution of the final epidemic size.

The basic reproduction number, R_0, is a little more difficult to describe. For this simple model R_0 is conveniently defined as the expected number of infections generated by one infectious individual in a large susceptible population. For the model presented above $R_0 = \lambda\iota$ since ι is the average length of the infectious period and during the infectious period an infectious individual has contact with initially susceptible individuals at rate λ. The branching approximation of Section 3.3 will in a rigorous way give the basic reproduction number the interpretation of a critical parameter indicating whether a large outbreak is possible or not. For epidemic models with different types of heterogeneities, it is not always obvious how R_0 should be defined. We shall return to this problem in Chapters 6 and 7.

2.2 The Sellke construction

The following alternative elegant construction of the standard SIR epidemic model is based on Sellke (1983). We keep track of the total 'infection pressure' generated by the infectious individuals. Each susceptible individual is associated with a critical level of 'exposure to infection', and as soon as the infection pressure reaches this level, the susceptible becomes infected. We call this level the *threshold* of the individual. This purely mathematical construction does not reflect any properties of a real-life epidemic but it will serve as an important tool in the derivation of several results in later chapters.

Label the initial infectives $-(m-1), -(m-2), \dots, 0$ and the initial susceptibles $1, 2, \dots, n$. Let $I_{-(m-1)}, I_{-(m-2)}, \dots, I_n$ be independent and identically distributed random variables, each distributed according to I. Also, let $Q_1, Q_2, \dots, Q_n$ be an independent sequence of independent and identically distributed exponential random variables, having mean 1. These are the individual thresholds. For $i = -(m-1), -(m-2), \dots, 0$, the initial infective labelled i remains infectious for a time I_i and is then removed. Denote by $Y(t)$ the number of infectives at time t, and let

$$A(t) = \frac{\lambda}{n} \int_0^t Y(u)\, du \tag{2.1}$$

be the total infection pressure exerted on a given susceptible up to time t. Note that in $A(t)$ the infectives are weighted according to their infectious periods. For $i = 1, 2, \dots, n$, the susceptible labelled i becomes infected when $A(t)$ reaches Q_i. The jth susceptible who becomes infected (*not* necessarily the susceptible labelled j!) remains infectious for a time I_j and is then removed. The epidemic ceases when there are no more infectives present.

In Figure 2.1 we have plotted the total infection pressure $A(t)$ against t for an epidemic starting with one infectious individual ($m = 1$). On the y-axis we have indicated the smallest individual thresholds ($Q_{(i)}$ denotes the ith order statistic) and horizontally the corresponding infectious period translated in time to the instant when the individual becomes infected. Note that the slope of $A(t)$ is proportional to the number of infectious periods covering the time point t (i.e. the number of infectives $Y(t)$!) as it should be according to the definition of A given in (2.1).

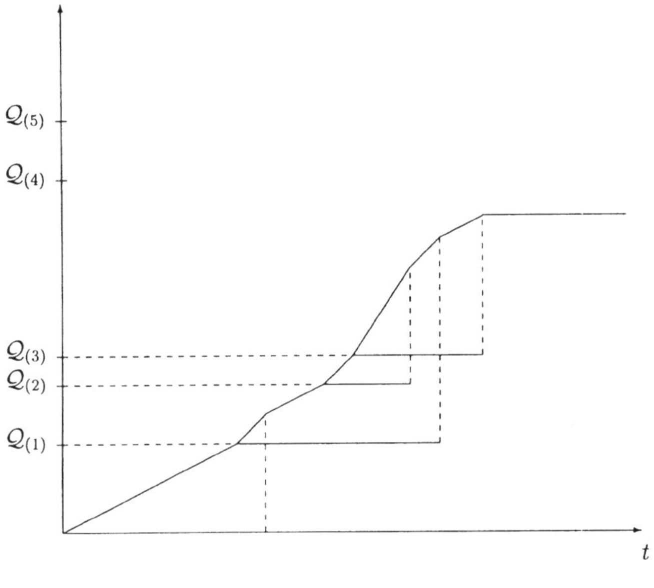

Figure 2.1: A typical realisation of the total infection pressure with $m = 1$ initially infectious individual. Note that the infection pressure never reaches $Q_{(4)}$ so the epidemic stops and the final size is $Z = 3$.

Let us check that this construction gives a process equivalent to the standard SIR epidemic. The infectious periods follow the correct distribution and, if $Y(t) = y$ and the individual labelled i is still susceptible at time t, then she will become infected during $(t, t + \Delta t)$ with probability $\lambda y \Delta t/n + o(\Delta t)$. Indeed, owing to the lack-of-memory property of the individual threshold Q_i, the probability of the complementary event is given by

$$\begin{aligned} \mathbf{P}(Q_i > A(t+\Delta t) \mid Q_i > A(t)) &= \mathbf{P}(Q_i > A(t+\Delta t) - A(t)) \\ &= e^{-[A(t+\Delta t)-A(t)]} \\ &= \exp\left(-\frac{\lambda}{n} y \Delta t + o(\Delta t)\right) \\ &= 1 - \lambda y \Delta t/n + o(\Delta t), \end{aligned}$$

where the third equality follows from the definition of $A(t)$, since no infections will occur in a small enough time increment, making $Y(u)$ constant and equal to y in $(t, t + \Delta t)$. In the original formulation of the model, our susceptible individual is contacted according to the superposition of y independent Poisson processes, each of intensity λ/n, giving rise to the same infection probability.

2.3 The Markovian case

Consider the standard SIR model $E_{n,m}(\lambda, I)$ and denote by $X(t)$ and $Y(t)$ the number of susceptibles and the number of infectives, respectively, at time t. The process $(X, Y) = \{(X(t), Y(t)); t \geq 0\}$ will be a Markov process if and only if the infectious period has the lack-of-memory property. Assume therefore that I is exponentially distributed with intensity γ. Then the process (X, Y) is governed by the following transition table:

from	to	at rate
(i, j)	$(i-1, j+1)$	$\lambda ij/n$
	$(i, j-1)$	γj

which follows immediately from the definition of the model. This model, which originated with Bartlett (1949), is known as the *general stochastic epidemic*, a name that now seems inappropriate, since the model has over the years been generalized in an innumerable number of ways. The assumption of an exponentially distributed infectious period is certainly not epidemiologically motivated, although with this assumption the mathematical analysis becomes much simpler. Notably, using Markov process theory we can obtain deterministic and diffusion approximations for the whole trajectory, which are valid for large population sizes (see Chapter 5). This is usually hard to achieve when the stochastic process is not Markovian. On the other hand, the modern probabilistic methods used in this text to derive branching process approximations (Section 3.3) together with results for the final epidemic size (Section

2.4 and Chapter 4) do *not* rely on the Markov property, but can be carried out for all instances of the standard SIR epidemic defined in Section 2.1.

2.4 Exact results

Consider again the standard SIR epidemic $E_{n,m}(\lambda, I)$. We will derive a triangular linear system of equations for $P^n = (P_0^n, P_1^n, \ldots, P_n^n)$, where P_k^n is the probability that k of the initial susceptibles are ultimately infected.

Let Z be the final size of the epidemic, and let $A = A(\infty) = \frac{\lambda}{n}\int_0^\infty Y(u)\,du$ be the total pressure of the epidemic. Recall the Sellke construction above. Both the final size and the total pressure can be expressed in terms of the infectious periods and the individual thresholds. First,

$$Z = \min\left\{ i : Q_{(i+1)} > \frac{\lambda}{n} \sum_{j=-(m-1)}^{i} I_j \right\},$$

where $Q_{(1)}, Q_{(2)}, \ldots, Q_{(n)}$ are the order statistics of $Q_1, Q_2, \ldots, Q_n$, since the epidemic stops as soon as the infection pressure generated by the previously infected individuals is insufficient to infect any more susceptibles. Also,

$$A = \frac{\lambda}{n} \sum_{j=-(m-1)}^{Z} I_j,$$

which is just another way of writing $A(\infty)$.

It is thus clear that the final size and the total pressure are intimately related. In fact, we have the following Wald's identity for epidemics (Ball, 1986):

Lemma 2.1 *Consider the standard SIR epidemic $E_{n,m}(\lambda, I)$ and let A be as above. Then*

$$E\left[e^{-\theta A}/\phi(\lambda\theta/n)^{Z+m}\right] = 1, \qquad \theta \geq 0,$$

where $\phi(\theta) = E[\exp(-\theta I)]$ is the Laplace transform of I.

Proof. To prove the identity, we note that

$$\begin{aligned}
\left(\phi(\lambda\theta/n)\right)^{n+m} &= E\left[\exp\left(-\frac{\lambda\theta}{n}\sum_{j=-(m-1)}^{n} I_j\right)\right] \\
&= E\left[\exp\left(-\theta\left(A + \frac{\lambda}{n}\sum_{j=Z+1}^{n} I_j\right)\right)\right] \\
&= E\left[e^{-\theta A}\left(\phi(\lambda\theta/n)\right)^{n-Z}\right],
\end{aligned}$$

where the last identity follows since the variables I_j, $j \geq Z+1$, are independent of both Z and A. •

We are now in position to derive the system of equations for $P^n = (P_0^n, \ldots, P_n^n)$. For each $k \geq 1$, define $\mathbf{K}$ to be the set $\{1, 2, \ldots, k\}$; also, let $\mathbf{0}$ be the empty set. Recall that the initial susceptibles are labelled $1, 2, \ldots, n$. P_k^n is the probability that k initial susceptibles are infected in the $E_{n,m}(\lambda, I)$ epidemic, and $P_{\mathbf{K}}^n$ is the probability that precisely the set $\mathbf{K}$ is infected. By symmetry, $P_k^n = \binom{n}{k} P_{\mathbf{K}}^n$.

Now fix k and choose ℓ such that $0 \leq k \leq \ell \leq n$, implying that $\mathbf{K} \subseteq \mathbf{L} \subseteq \mathbf{N}$. We use the notion of infection pressure to compare an epidemic within $\mathbf{N}$ with a sub-epidemic within $\mathbf{L}$. The event that an epidemic within $\mathbf{N}$ infects precisely the set $\mathbf{K}$ is the same as the event that a sub-epidemic within $\mathbf{L}$ infects precisely $\mathbf{K}$, and that these k new infectives, together with the m initial infectives, fail to infect any of the individuals in the set $\mathbf{N} \setminus \mathbf{L}$. We know from the Sellke construction that the probability of avoiding the infection is given by $\exp(-a)$, given that the sub-epidemic has generated the infection pressure $A^\ell = a$. It follows that

$$P_{\mathbf{K}}^n = P_{\mathbf{K}}^\ell E[\exp(-A^\ell(n-\ell)) \mid Z^\ell = k],$$

where Z^ℓ is the final size of the sub-epidemic. This equation is equivalent to

$$\frac{\binom{\ell}{k} P_k^n}{\binom{n}{k}} = P_k^\ell E[\exp(-A^\ell(n-\ell)) \mid Z^\ell = k]. \tag{2.2}$$

Now let us use Wald's identity (Lemma 2.1) applied to the sub-epidemic and with $\theta = n - \ell$ to get

$$E\left[e^{-A^\ell(n-\ell)} / [\phi(\lambda(n-\ell)/n)]^{Z^\ell+m}\right] = 1,$$

or, conditioning on the final size Z^ℓ,

$$\sum_{k=0}^{\ell} \frac{P_k^\ell E\left(\exp(-A^\ell(n-\ell)) \mid Z^\ell = k\right)}{[\phi(\lambda(n-\ell)/n)]^{k+m}} = 1. \tag{2.3}$$

Equations (2.2) and (2.3) immediately give us

$$\sum_{k=0}^{\ell} \frac{\binom{\ell}{k} P_k^n}{\binom{n}{k} [\phi(\lambda(n-\ell)/n)]^{k+m}} = 1.$$

Finally, noting that $\binom{\ell}{k} / \binom{n}{k} = \binom{n-k}{\ell-k} / \binom{n}{\ell}$, we arrive at the following result:

Theorem 2.2 *Consider the standard SIR epidemic $E_{n,m}(\lambda, I)$. Denote by P_k^n the probability that the final size of the epidemic is equal to k, $0 \leq k \leq n$. Then*

$$\sum_{k=0}^{\ell} \binom{n-k}{\ell-k} P_k^n / [\phi(\lambda(n-\ell)/n)]^{k+m} = \binom{n}{\ell}, \qquad 0 \leq \ell \leq n. \tag{2.4}$$

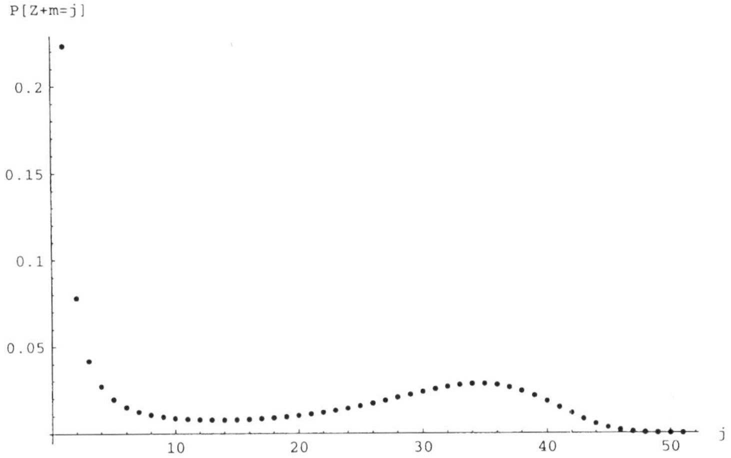

Figure 2.2: The exact distribution of $Z + m$ for $m = 1$, $n = 50$, $\lambda = 1.5$ and $I \equiv 1$, i.e. the infectious period is constant and equal to 1.

Note that, since the system of equations is triangular, the final-size-probabilities can be solved recursively. The proof of the theorem depends on the *infection pressure* generated by the various infectives, rather than the actual infectious periods. This indicates that we may allow for latent periods and time-dependent infection rates in the modelling, and still get the same type of final size results, as long as the required infection pressure can be calculated. That this is indeed the case will become even clearer in Section 7.1 where the concept of random graphs is used to describe the epidemic flow through a homogeneous and uniformly mixing population. In Figure 2.2 the probabilities $P_0^n, P_1^n, \ldots, P_n^n$, are plotted for a specific choice of community and parameter values (the figure actually shows the plot of $P(Z + m = k)$ for different values of k but since $m = 1$ this corresponds to P_{k-1}^n). When the infectious period is constant, $I \equiv c$ say, an infectious individual infects susceptible individuals independently (with probability $p = 1 - e^{-\lambda c}$); the distribution of the final size is then equivalent to the Reed-Frost model defined for discrete time dynamics in Section 1.2. It is seen in the figure that the distribution is bimodal: either a few individuals are infected or else a fairly large number are infected. This qualitative behavior becomes more and more evident as n, the initial number of susceptibles, increases. A mathematical proof ofthis is given by the threshold limit theorem of Chapter 4.

Finally we mention briefly the very elegant theory developed by Lefèvre and Picard in a series of papers (see e.g. Lefèvre and Picard, 1990). They work with quite general classes of stochastic epidemic models, both single-type and multitype (cf. Chapter 6), and derive e.g. equations for the final size distribution and the total force of infection

$A(\infty)$, using a non-standard family of polynomials initially introduced by Gontcharoff (1937). However, we have decided not to include any presentation of their work, since the approach is rather algebraic in nature, and hardly increases the intuitive understanding of the models treated here.

Exercises

2.1. Compute P_0^n, P_1^n and P_2^n numerically using the recursive formula given by (2.4) assuming $n = 10$, $m = 1$, $\lambda = 2$ and that the infectious period I is:

a) exponentially distributed (the Markovian case) with mean 1 time unit.

b) $\Gamma(2, 2)$-distributed (i.e. with mean 1).

c) constant and equal to 1.

2.2. Assume $m = 1$, $\lambda = 1$ and that the infectious period is constant with mean 1 time unit. Use your favorite computer and mathematical software to see when the recursive formula of Section 2.4 breaks down numerically by computing and plotting $P_1^n, \ldots, P_n^n$ for $n = 10, 20, 30, \ldots$ (for most computers negative probabilities start appearing around $n \approx 70 - 90$).

2.3. Modify the standard SIR epidemic so that the infectious period is $= \infty$. (This model is denoted the SI model since individuals never get removed. It also has applications in sociology for the spread of rumours/knowledge. Infectious then corresponds to knowing, and spreading, the rumour.) For this model $X(t) + Y(t) = n + m$ for all t. Assume $m = 1$. Describe the random process $Y = \{Y(t); t \geq 0\}$, of infectious individuals. Calculate the expected waiting time until everyone in the population becomes infected. (Hint: Consider the consecutive waiting times between infections.) What happens with this expression when n gets large?

3 Coupling methods

Let us assume that we are interested in comparing two or more random elements with each other. It is sometimes possible to construct versions of these random elements on the same probability space, in such a way that the comparison suddenly becomes easy (indeed, often trivial) to carry out. This procedure is called *coupling*, the term referring to the fact that the random elements so constructed are often highly dependent. The coupling method has found many important applications in various fields of probability theory, including Markov processes, renewal processes and Poisson approximation. The book by Lindvall (1992) provides a nice introduction to the subject.

Here we introduce some classical coupling ideas by providing simple examples. Then, after presenting the formal definition, we describe some applications of the coupling method to the standard SIR epidemic model $E_{n,m}(\lambda, I)$. First, it is shown that the number of infectious individuals in a large population initially behaves like a branching process. By coupling $E_{n,m}(\lambda, I)$ with a branching process, we justify the approximation of the epidemic by the simpler and thoroughly analysed branching process. This result indicates at the same time the significance of the basic reproduction number R_0. Second, by coupling two epidemics with different contact parameter λ, we prove the intuitively obvious fact that the accumulated number of infected individuals at a given time grows (in a sense yet to be defined) with λ, the infectiousness of the disease.

3.1 First examples

Gambler's ruin problem

Consider first the standard gambler's ruin problem. An individual with an initial capital of m units of money goes to a casino. He plays a series of independent games, in each of which he wins one unit with probability θ and loses one unit with probability $1 - \theta$. He continues until either his capital reaches n ($n > m$) or he goes bankrupt. We wish to use coupling to prove that $P(\theta)$, the probability of reaching the capital n given θ, is increasing in θ (as would be expected).

To this end, let $U_1, U_2, \dots$ be independent and identically distributed random variables, each uniformly distributed on the interval $(0, 1)$. Then, for a given θ, define

$$Y_\theta(i) = \begin{cases} +1 & \text{if } U_i \leq \theta, \\ -1 & \text{otherwise,} \end{cases}$$

$i = 1, 2, \dots,$ and

$$X_\theta(\nu) = m + \sum_{i=1}^{\nu} Y_\theta(i),$$

$\nu = 1, 2, \ldots$. Then, since $Y_\theta(i)$ is $+1$ with probability θ, the process $X_\theta = \{X_\theta(\nu); \nu = 1, 2, \ldots\}$, clearly describes the capital of the gambler. Note carefully that the *same* set of uniform variables is used to construct an entire family of trajectories, indexed by θ. Now, if $\theta < \theta'$ then by construction $Y_\theta(i) \leq Y_{\theta'}(i)$ for all i, so $X_\theta(\nu) \leq X_{\theta'}(\nu)$ for all ν. This means that if a trajectory $X_\theta(\nu)$ reaches n before 0 then the same is true for $X_{\theta'}(\nu)$. Thus we have that $P(\theta) \leq P(\theta')$, since this property does not depend on the particular sample space chosen.

Stochastic ordering

Let X and X' be real-valued random variables. We say that X is *stochastically smaller* than X' and write $X \overset{\mathcal{D}}{\leq} X'$ if

$$\mathbf{P}(X \geq a) \leq \mathbf{P}(X' \geq a)$$

for all a, i.e. the probability that X exceeds an arbitrary level is smaller than the probability that X' exceeds the same level.

When working with stochastically ordered random variables, the following simple result can often be very helpful: if X and X' are random variables such that $X \overset{\mathcal{D}}{\leq} X'$, then there exists a coupling $(\hat{X}, \hat{X}')$ of X and X' such that $\hat{X} \leq \hat{X}'$. The proof goes as follows. For a given distribution function G, define the generalized inverse G^* of G by

$$G^*(u) = \inf\{x : G(x) \geq u\}, \qquad 0 < u < 1.$$

Then $G^*(U)$ has distribution function G if U is uniformly distributed on $(0, 1)$. If F and F' are the distribution functions of X and X', respectively, we have $F \geq F'$ by assumption. Thus $F^* \leq F'^*$, and we see that the variables $\hat{X} = F^*(U)$ and $\hat{X}' = F'^*(U)$ provide us with the desired coupling.

Domination of birth and death processes

In our next example, different birth and death processes are compared. Suppose that $X = \{X(t); t \geq 0\}$, and $X' = \{X'(t); t \geq 0\}$, are two birth and death processes on the set of nonnegative integers. The process X has birth rates λ_i and death rates μ_i,

$$\begin{aligned} \mathbf{P}(X(t+dt) - X(t) = +1 \mid X(t) = i) &= \lambda_i dt + o(dt), \\ \mathbf{P}(X(t+dt) - X(t) = -1 \mid X(t) = i) &= \mu_i dt + o(dt), \end{aligned}$$

$X(0) = m$, and likewise X' has birth rates λ_i', death rates μ_i' and initial value m'. We use coupling to show that if $\lambda_i \leq \lambda_i'$ for all $i \geq 0$ and $\mu_i \geq \mu_i'$ for all $i \geq 1$ then $X(t)$ is stochastically smaller than $X'(t)$ for all t (provided also $m \leq m'$).

Define a bivariate process $(\hat{X}, \hat{X}')$ with initial value (m, m') and with the following intensity table:

from	to	at rate
(i,j)	$(i+1,j)$	λ_i
	$(i,j+1)$	λ'_j
	$(i-1,j)$	μ_i
	$(i,j-1)$	μ'_j
(i,i)	$(i+1,i+1)$	λ_i
	$(i,i+1)$	$\lambda'_i - \lambda_i$
	$(i-1,i-1)$	μ'_i
	$(i-1,i)$	$\mu_i - \mu'_i$.

This process is well-defined since all the numbers describing the transition rates are nonnegative by assumption. It is easily checked that the first coordinate $\hat{X}$ follows the same law as X. Likewise, the second coordinate is distributed as X'. Moreover, if the bivariate process starts above the diagonal $i = j$ then it will stay above the diagonal at all times. Hence we have found versions $\hat{X}$ and $\hat{X}'$ with $\hat{X}(t) \leq \hat{X}'(t)$ for all t; in particular $X(t) \overset{\mathcal{D}}{\leq} X'(t)$ for all t, since this latter property has nothing to do with the sample space chosen.

Convergence of Markov chains

As a final illustration of the coupling method we show the classical result that an irreducible aperiodic Markov chain with a finite m-state space approaches stationarity as time grows, regardless of the initial distribution. Let $X = (X(0), X(1), \dots)$ be such a Markov chain and denote its transition probability matrix by P and its initial distribution by λ. Also, let $\pi = (\pi_1, \dots, \pi_m)$ be the unique strictly positive stationary distribution, satisfying $\pi = \pi P$. We wish to prove that $\mathbf{P}(X(\nu) = j) \to \pi_j$ as $\nu \to \infty$, for all fixed states j, $j = 1, \dots, m$.

We now give the classical coupling proof. Introduce a Markov chain $X' = (X'(0), X'(1), \dots)$, independent of X, governed by the transition matrix P, and with initial distribution π. This makes X' stationary. Then fix a state j and define $\hat{X} = (\hat{X}(0), \hat{X}(1), \dots)$ by

$$\hat{X}(\nu) = \begin{cases} X(\nu) & \text{if } \nu < T, \\ X'(\nu) & \text{if } \nu \geq T, \end{cases}$$

where

$$T = \min\{\nu \geq 0 : X(\nu) = X'(\nu)\}.$$

Due to the (strong) Markov property, the processes $\hat{X}$ and X will be equally distributed. Thus

$$|\mathbf{P}(X(\nu) = j) - \mathbf{P}(X'(\nu) = j)| = |\mathbf{P}(\hat{X}(\nu) = j) - \mathbf{P}(X'(\nu) = j)|$$

$$= |\mathbf{P}(\hat{X}(\nu) = j, T > \nu) - \mathbf{P}(X'(\nu) = j, T > \nu)| \leq \mathbf{P}(T > \nu).$$

It is easy to see that $\mathbf{P}(T > \nu) \to 0$ as $\nu \to \infty$, i.e. that T is finite a.s. Indeed, the bivariate process (X, X') is irreducible and aperiodic, and T is the first time this process visits the diagonal.

3.2 Definition of coupling

Skills in coupling are acquired only by working through many examples. The actual definition is not very illuminating, but we give it here anyway for the sake of completeness. Given probability spaces $(\Omega, \mathcal{F}, \mathbf{P})$ and $(\Omega', \mathcal{F}', \mathbf{P}')$, denote the state space by E; E could be the set of nonnegative integers, the set of real numbers, the set of sequences of real numbers, the space of right-continuous real-valued functions defined on $[0, \infty)$, and so on.

By a *coupling* of the random elements $X : \Omega \to E$ and $X' : \Omega' \to E$ we mean a probability space $(\hat{\Omega}, \hat{\mathcal{F}}, \hat{\mathbf{P}})$ and a random element $(\hat{X}, \hat{X}') : \hat{\Omega} \to E^2$ such that

$$X \stackrel{\mathcal{D}}{=} \hat{X} \qquad \text{and} \qquad X' \stackrel{\mathcal{D}}{=} \hat{X}'.$$

In our first example, the desired result was obtained by putting $\hat{X} = X_\theta$ and $\hat{X}' = X_{\theta'}$. The second and third example also fit nicely into our definition, and so does the last one if we put $\hat{X}' = X'$.

3.3 Applications to epidemics

Initial approximation

Intuitively speaking, during the initial stages of an epidemic in a large population we would expect that, with high probability, contacted individuals are susceptible, so that the number of infectious individuals follows some kind of branching behaviour. This branching approximation idea has a long history, see e.g. Bartlett (1955) and Kendall (1956). Here, following Ball and Donnelly (1995), we use a coupling argument to investigate how the approximation improves as the population size tends to infinity.

Let us first define the branching process, and derive heuristically some initial results concerning this process. At time $t = 0$ there exists a group of m ancestors (that have just been born). The life spans of different individuals are independent and identically distributed according to a random variable I. During her life span, a given ancestor gives birth at the time points of a Poisson process with intensity λ. Her children have independent and identically distributed life spans and themselves give birth according to Poisson processes with intensity λ, and so on. We assume that all Poisson processes are independent of each other; they are also independent of the life spans. Denote the resulting process by $E_m(\lambda, I)$. Jagers (1975) gives a thorough treatment of a class of continuous time branching processes containing the above process as a special case.

Let $\{Y(t); t \geq 0\}$, be the number of individuals alive at time t, $t \geq 0$, and denote by D the number of offspring of a given individual. We wish to investigate the possible extinction/explosion of $Y(t)$ as t grows. First, since there are on the average $mE(D)^\nu$ individuals in the νth generation, it is intuitively clear that the process will become extinct if and only $E(D) \leq 1$. Turning to the more interesting case where $E(D) > 1$, we let q be the extinction probability of the branching process and first assume that $m = 1$. Then, by letting D_0 be the number of children of the ancestor, we have

$$q = \sum_{k=0}^{\infty} \mathbf{P}(\text{extinction} \mid D_0 = k)\mathbf{P}(D_0 = k).$$

But ultimate extinction will occur if and only if all of the (independent) branches generated by these children become extinct, hence $q = \sum_{k=0}^{\infty} q^k \mathbf{P}(D_0 = k)$, showing that q is the solution of the equation $\theta = E(\theta^D)$. With a little more work one can show that q is the *smallest* solution to this equation. Finally, when there are m ancestors the extinction probability is given by q^m with q as above. For detailed proofs of all these results, see Jagers (1975).

We conclude our description of the process $E_m(\lambda, I)$ by presenting the fundamental quantities encountered above in a somewhat more explicit form. Note that, given $I = t$, the number of children D is Poisson distributed with mean λt. It follows that the probability generating function of D is

$$\begin{aligned} E(\theta^D) &= E\left(E(\theta^D \mid I)\right) \\ &= E\left(\exp\{-\lambda I(1-\theta)\}\right) \\ &= \phi(\lambda(1-\theta)), \end{aligned}$$

and its expectation is

$$E(D) = \lambda \iota,$$

where the probability generating function and the expectation of I are given by ϕ and ι, respectively. Also note that the variance of D is strictly positive, even if the lifetime I is constant.

Returning to the main topic of this section, we examine the branching approximation of our epidemic process. Consider a sequence of standard SIR epidemic processes $E_{n,m}(\lambda, I)$, $n \geq 1$. Let $\{Y_n(t); t \geq 0\}$, be the process describing the number of infectives in the nth epidemic. We wish to compare this process with $\{Y(t); t \geq 0\}$, the process describing the number of individuals alive in the continuous time branching process $E_m(\lambda, I)$.

First we construct the branching process $E_m(\lambda, I)$. Suppose that the probability space $(\Omega, \mathcal{F}, \mathbf{P})$ holds the individual life histories $\mathcal{H}_{-(m-1)}, \mathcal{H}_{-(m-2)}, \ldots,$ where each

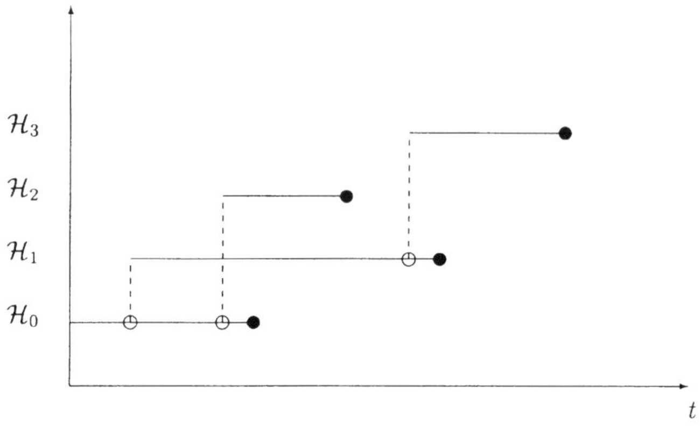

Figure 3.1: Construction of $E_m(\lambda, I)$ for $m = 1$ using life histories.

$\mathcal{H}_i$ is a list containing the life span of the ith individual together with the time points at which this individual gives birth. Let $\mathcal{H}_{-(m-1)}, \mathcal{H}_{-(m-2)}, \dots, \mathcal{H}_0$ be the life histories of the m ancestors and let $\mathcal{H}_i$, $i \geq 1$, be the life history of the ith individual born.

Next, we use an independent sequence U_i, $i \geq 1$, of independent and identically distributed random variables defined on $(\Omega, \mathcal{F}, \mathbf{P})$, each uniformly distributed on $(0, 1)$, to construct all of the epidemic processes $E_{n,m}(\lambda, I)$, $n \geq 1$. Fix n and label the initial susceptibles $1, 2, \dots, n$. The initial ancestors in the branching process correspond to the initial infectives in the epidemic. A contact in the epidemic process occurs whenever a birth occurs in the branching process. The individual contacted at the ith contact has label $C_i = [nU_i] + 1$. If this individual is still susceptible, then she becomes infected in the epidemic, otherwise she and all of her descendants in the branching process are ignored in the epidemic process. In the latter case the individual is called a *ghost*, following Mollison (1977). Finally, the death of an non-ghost individual in the branching process corresponds to removal in the epidemic. This construction leads to a process equivalent to $E_{n,m}(\lambda, I)$.

In Figure 3.1 the construction of $E_m(\lambda, I)$ is illustrated with $m = 1$. The life histories of the initially infectious individuals are inserted horizontally one at each y-level, starting at $t = 0$ (in the example only $\mathcal{H}_0$ since $m = 1$). As t grows, a new life history is inserted whenever there is a birth among the life histories present. In the construction of the epidemic $E_{n,m}(\lambda, I)$ the same procedure is used, except that the life history is not inserted if the label C_i has appeared previously, i.e. the individual is a ghost.

Obviously, the processes Y_n and Y agree until the time T_n of the first ghost. The number of births in the branching process during a fixed time interval $[0, t_0]$ is finite a.s. It is easily checked that any finite number of labels C_i will be distinct with a probability tending to 1 as $n \to \infty$, showing that

$$\mathbf{P}(T_n > t_0) \to 1 \qquad \text{as } n \to \infty.$$

Ball and Donnelly (1995) have shown that the branching process breaks down roughly at time $C \log(n)$. Note that the problem of deciding the number of contacts made before a previously infected individual is picked again, i.e. the number of trials before one of the labels C_i is repeated, is a variant of the classical birthday problem.

We collect our findings in the following theorem:

Theorem 3.1 *Consider a sequence of epidemic processes $E_{n,m}(\lambda, I)$, $n \geq 1$. Also, denote by $Y_n(t)$ the number of infectives at time t, $t \geq 0$. Then, for each fixed t_0, $Y_n(t_0) \to Y(t_0)$ almost surely, where $\{Y(t); t \geq 0\}$, is the process describing the number of individuals alive in the branching process $E_m(\lambda, I)$.*

If $\lambda\iota \leq 1$ then Y becomes extinct with probability 1. On the other hand, if $\lambda\iota > 1$ then Y becomes extinct with probability q^m, where q is the smallest root of the equation $\phi(\lambda(1-\theta)) = \theta$, or explodes with probability $1 - q^m$.

This result shows that the basic reproduction number $R_0 = \lambda\iota$ determines, for a large population, whether or not a large outbreak of the epidemic may occur.

Monotonicity

We finally show how coupling can be used to compare epidemics with the same distribution for infectious periods but with different infection rates. We consider two standard SIR epidemic models $E_{n,m}(\lambda, I)$ and $E_{n,m}(\lambda', I)$ where $\lambda \leq \lambda'$, and prove that the accumulated number of infected individuals at time t for the epidemic with infection rate λ is stochastically smaller than the corresponding quantity for the epidemic with rate λ'.

Let us return to the Sellke construction. Let $I_{-(m-1)}, I_{-(m-2)}, \ldots, I_n$ be the infectious periods and let $Q_1, Q_2, \ldots, Q_n$ be the individual thresholds of the epidemic $E_{n,m}(\lambda, I)$. Thus the variables Q_i, $1 \leq i \leq n$, are exponentially distributed with intensity 1. To construct $E_{n,m}(\lambda', I)$, use the *same* realizations of infectious periods and individual thresholds. Only the infection pressure processes, $A(t)$ and $A'(t)$, respectively, are different for the two models.

For $1 \leq j \leq n$, define T_j to be the time of the jth infection in the epidemic with infection rate λ; $T_j = \infty$ if the final size is strictly less than j. Similarly define T'_j, $1 \leq j \leq n$, for the epidemic process with infection rate λ'. The first infection in the epidemic with rate λ' will occur earlier than the first infection in the other epidemic, i.e. $T_1' \leq T_1$, since $A(t) \leq A'(t)$ up to the time point T_1'. This will give rise to an even larger difference in magnitude between the two infection pressure processes. Consequently, it follows that $T_2' \leq T_2$, and so on. The desired result follows, since

$$|\{j : T_j \leq t\}| \leq |\{j : T_j' \leq t\}|$$

for all t.

Exercises

3.1. Check that the process $(\hat{X}, \hat{X}')$, defined in the section on domination of birth and death processes, is indeed a coupling of the birth and death processes X and X', i.e. that the marginal distributions coincide with the distributions of X and X', respectively.

3.2. In Section 3.3 we saw that the branching approximation broke down on the part of the sample space where the size of the total progeny in the branching process was infinite. Show that in this case the first ghost in the construction appears when approximately $\sqrt{n}$ individuals have become infected. It is well-known in branching process theory that, given explosion, the total number born before t grows like $e^{\alpha t}$, where α (the so-called Malthusian parameter) satisfies a certain equation. What can hence be said about the *time* of the appearance of the first ghost?

3.3. Consider the Markovian version (Section 2.3) of the standard SIR epidemic (m fixed, n large). Without referring to the branching approximation of Section 3.3, approximate the process of infectives $Y_n(t)$ during the initial stage of the epidemic with a suitable simple birth and death process. What is the probability of extinction/explosion of this approximating process? (Hint: $X_n(t) \approx n$ during the initial stage of the epidemic.)

4 The threshold limit theorem

We will now explore in greater detail the large population limit of the final size distribution for the standard SIR epidemic model $E_{n,m}(\lambda, I)$. We have seen (Section 3.3) that, if the population of susceptibles is large and we introduce a small number of initial infectives, the number of infectious individuals behaves like a branching process in the beginning. If the basic reproduction number $R_0 = \lambda\iota$ is less than or equal to 1, a small outbreak will occur. On the other hand, if R_0 exceeds 1, then there is a positive probability that the approximating branching process explodes; this implies, of course, that the branching process approximation will break down after some time. Then it is reasonable to expect that the final epidemic size will satisfy a law of large numbers. This indicates that the asymptotic distribution of the final size actually consists of two parts, one close to zero and the other concentrated around some deterministic value. In this chapter we sketch the derivation of these results, using the Sellke construction and the beautiful imbedding representation of Scalia-Tomba (1985, 1990). A fluctuation result for the final size, given a large outbreak, will also be given. In the final section we combine earlier results and indicate the proof of a theorem due to Barbour (1975) on the duration of the (Markovian) standard SIR epidemic.

4.1 The imbedded process

To explain the imbedding idea, we need to introduce two auxiliary processes; the infection pressure process

$$\mathcal{I}(t) = \frac{\lambda}{n} \sum_{j=-(m-1)}^{[t]-m} I_j, \qquad 0 \le t \le n+m,$$

and the threshold process

$$\mathcal{Q}(t) = \sum_{j=1}^{n} \mathbf{1}_{\{Q_j \le t\}}, \qquad t \ge 0.$$

Recall that the variables I_j are the infectious periods, and the variables Q_j are the individual thresholds. The index t should *not* be interpreted as ordinary time.

We know from Section 2.4 that the final size Z can be written

$$Z = \min\left\{ i \ge 0 \,:\, Q_{(i+1)} > \frac{\lambda}{n} \sum_{j=-(m-1)}^{i} I_j \right\}.$$

Let us express this quantity in terms of the infectivity and the susceptibility processes. By definition, $Z = i$ if and only if

$$\begin{aligned} Q_{(1)} &\leq \mathcal{I}(0+m), \\ Q_{(2)} &\leq \mathcal{I}(1+m), \\ &\vdots \\ Q_{(i)} &\leq \mathcal{I}(i-1+m), \\ Q_{(i+1)} &> \mathcal{I}(i+m). \end{aligned}$$

Put another way, the pressure $\mathcal{I}(0+m)$ is enough to infect at least one individual, the pressure $\mathcal{I}(1+m)$ is then enough to infect at least two individuals, and so on. Hence

$$\begin{aligned} \mathcal{Q}(\mathcal{I}(0+m)) &> 0, \\ \mathcal{Q}(\mathcal{I}(1+m)) &> 1, \\ &\vdots \\ \mathcal{Q}(\mathcal{I}(i-1+m)) &> i-1, \\ \mathcal{Q}(\mathcal{I}(i+m)) &\leq i. \end{aligned}$$

It follows immediately that

$$Z = \min\{t \geq 0 \, : \, \mathcal{Q}(\mathcal{I}(t+m)) = t\}.$$

For future use, denote the composition $\mathcal{Q}(\mathcal{I}(t))$ by $\mathcal{C}(t)$. Figure 4.1 shows simulated realizations of $\mathcal{C}(t)$ for two different population sizes. The final size Z is the "time" when $\mathcal{C}(t)$ intersects t.

4.2 Preliminary convergence results

From now on we consider a sequence of epidemic processes $E_{n,m}(\lambda, I)$, $n \geq 1$; the quantities defined above will now have a subscript n. It is straightforward to analyse the (independent!) processes $\mathcal{I}_n$ and $\mathcal{Q}_n$. Define $\bar{\mathcal{I}}_n(t) = \mathcal{I}_n(nt)$ and $\bar{\mathcal{Q}}_n(t) = \mathcal{Q}_n(t)/n$. Then

$$\bar{\mathcal{I}}_n(t) \to \lambda\iota t \qquad \text{and} \qquad \bar{\mathcal{Q}}_n(t) \to 1 - e^{-t}$$

in probability, uniformly on compact sets. Here we recall that $\iota = E(I)$. Since composition is a continuous operation, it follows that

$$\bar{\mathcal{C}}_n(t) = \bar{\mathcal{Q}}_n(\bar{\mathcal{I}}_n(t)) \to 1 - e^{-\lambda\iota t}$$

in probability, uniformly on compact sets. We also have the following fluctuation results. The sequence of processes

$$\sqrt{n}\left(\bar{\mathcal{I}}_n(t) - \lambda\iota t\right), \quad t \geq 0,$$

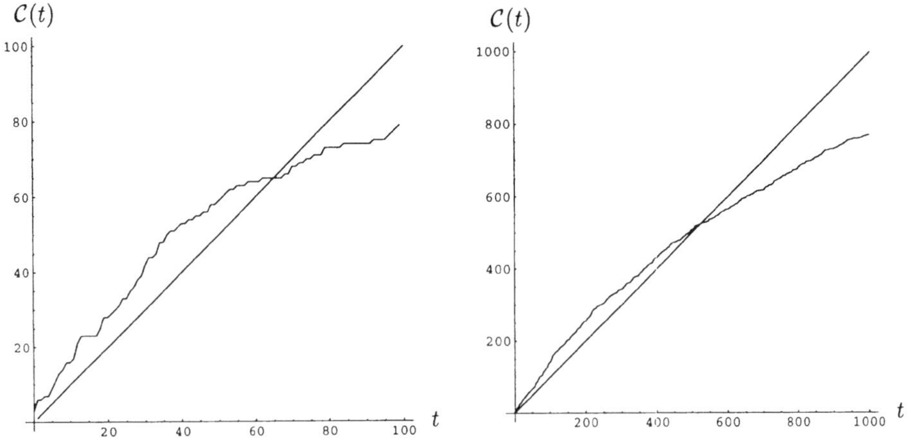

Figure 4.1: Simulation of the imbedded process $\mathcal{C}(t)$ for $n = 100$ (left) and $n = 1000$ (right).

$n \geq 1$, converges in distribution to a Wiener process with variance $\lambda^2\sigma^2 t$. Also, the sequence

$$\sqrt{n}\left(\bar{\mathcal{Q}}_n(t) - \left[1 - e^{-t}\right]\right), \quad t \geq 0,$$

$n \geq 1$, converges weakly to a Gaussian process with mean 0 and variance $e^{-t}\left(1 - e^{-t}\right)$. (Readers not familiar with the theory of weak convergence of sequences of random processes may consult e.g. Billingsley, 1968. Convergence for a *fixed* arbitrary value of t follows from the usual law of large numbers and the central limit theorem, hence the stated results are certainly plausible.) Finally, in order to study the fluctuations $\tilde{\mathcal{C}}_n(t)$ of the composite process $\mathcal{C}_n(t) = \mathcal{Q}_n(\mathcal{I}_n(t))$ we write

$$\begin{aligned}\sqrt{n}\left(\bar{\mathcal{Q}}_n(\bar{\mathcal{I}}_n(t)) - \left[1 - e^{-\lambda\iota t}\right]\right) &= \sqrt{n}\left(\bar{\mathcal{Q}}_n(\bar{\mathcal{I}}_n(t)) - \left[1 - e^{-\bar{\mathcal{I}}_n(t)}\right]\right) \\ &+ \sqrt{n}\left(\left[1 - e^{-\bar{\mathcal{I}}_n(t)}\right] - \left[1 - e^{-\lambda\iota t}\right]\right).\end{aligned}$$

It is seen that this process converges weakly to a zero mean Gaussian process $\tilde{\mathcal{C}}(t)$ with variance

$$e^{-\lambda\iota t}\left(1 - e^{-\lambda\iota t}\right) + \lambda^2\sigma^2 t e^{-2\lambda\iota t}.$$

All of the results above are derived rigorously by Scalia-Tomba (1985, 1990).

4.3 The case $m_n/n \to \mu > 0$ as $n \to \infty$

Write the final size proportion as

$$\frac{Z_n}{n} = \frac{1}{n}\min\left\{t \geq 0 : \bar{C}_n\left(\frac{t}{n} + \frac{m_n}{n}\right) = \frac{t}{n}\right\}.$$

Working with $Z_n' = Z_n + m_n$, which includes the initial infectives in the final size, will lead to cleaner formulas. We know that $\bar{C}_n(t)$ converges in probability to $1 - e^{-\lambda\iota t}$, and also that $m_n/n \to \mu > 0$ by assumption. It is thus easily seen that the sequence $\bar{Z}_n' = Z_n'/n$ converges to τ, the unique solution to the equation

$$1 - e^{-\lambda\iota\tau} = \tau - \mu.$$

To give an intuitive explanation of this equation, rewrite it as

$$1 + \mu - \tau = e^{-\lambda\iota\tau}. \tag{4.1}$$

A given individual avoids becoming infected by a given infective with probability $E\left(e^{-\lambda I/n}\right)$. Hence the probability of escaping infection is given by

$$\left[E\left(e^{-\lambda I/n}\right)\right]^{Z_n'} \approx \left(1 - \frac{\lambda\iota}{n}\right)^{n\tau} \approx e^{-\lambda\iota\tau},$$

i.e. the right hand side of (4.1). But the probability of escaping infection is of course equal to the proportion of initial susceptibles who remain uninfected, i.e. the left hand side of (4.1).

In Figure 4.2 the two functions $f(t) = 1 + \mu - t$ and $g(t) = e^{-\lambda\iota t}$ are plotted for the case $\mu = 0.1$, $\lambda = 1.8$ and $\iota = 1$. The intersection of the two curves defines the unique solution $\tau \approx 0.903$.

To obtain a central limit theorem for Z_n', we proceed as follows. Since $\bar{Z}_n' = \bar{C}_n(\bar{Z}_n') + m_n/n$ and $\tau = 1 - e^{-\lambda\iota\tau} + \mu$, we may write

$$\begin{aligned}
\sqrt{n}\left(\bar{Z}_n' - \tau\right) &= \sqrt{n}\left(\bar{C}_n\left(\bar{Z}_n'\right) - \left[1 - e^{-\lambda\iota\bar{Z}_n'}\right]\right) \\
&+ \sqrt{n}\left(\left[1 - e^{-\lambda\iota\bar{Z}_n'}\right] - \left[1 - e^{-\lambda\iota\tau}\right]\right) + o(1) \\
&= \sqrt{n}\left(\bar{C}_n\left(\bar{Z}_n'\right) - \left[1 - e^{-\lambda\iota\bar{Z}_n'}\right]\right) \\
&+ \lambda\iota e^{-\lambda\iota\tau}\sqrt{n}\left(\bar{Z}_n' - \tau\right) + o(1).
\end{aligned}$$

Rearranging and taking limits yields that the sequence $\sqrt{n}(\bar{Z}_n' - \tau)$ converges to a normally distributed random variable with mean 0 and variance

$$\left(e^{-\lambda\iota\tau}\left(1 - e^{-\lambda\iota\tau}\right) + \lambda^2\sigma^2\tau e^{-2\lambda\iota\tau}\right) / \left(1 - \lambda\iota e^{-\lambda\iota\tau}\right)^2.$$

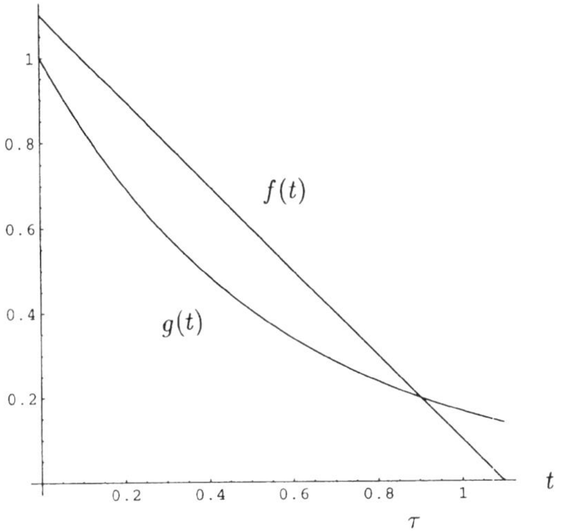

Figure 4.2: Graphical illustration of τ, the solution to (4.1), for $\mu = 0.1$, $\lambda = 1.8$ and $\iota = 1$.

The expression above is well-defined if the condition

$$\lambda\iota e^{-\lambda\iota\tau} < 1$$

is fulfilled. To see that this is indeed the case, consider the functions $\exp(-\lambda\iota t)$ and $1 + \mu - t$ in Figure 4.2. The derivative of the exponential function has to be strictly greater than -1 at the crossing point τ, leading to the desired conclusion. The condition has actually a very natural interpretation. At the beginning, the basic reproduction number is given by $R_0 = \lambda\iota$, i.e. an infectious individual generates on the average $\lambda\iota$ new cases in a large susceptible population. However, after a large outbreak a fraction $1 - (\tau - \mu)$ has escaped infection so that a second introduction of the disease in the population would correspond to the effective basic reproduction number $\lambda\iota(1 - (\tau - \mu)) = \lambda\iota\exp(-\lambda\iota\tau)$. This number is less than 1, otherwise the epidemic would not have ceased in the first place.

Let us state our results as a theorem.

Theorem 4.1 *Consider a sequence of epidemic processes $E_{n,m_n}(\lambda, I)$. Assume that $m_n/n \to \mu > 0$ as $n \to \infty$ and define τ as the solution to (4.1). Also denote the final epidemic size by Z_n and write $Z_n' = Z_n + m_n$. Then the sequence $\sqrt{n}(Z_n'/n - \tau)$ converges to a normally distributed random variable with mean 0 and variance*

$$\frac{\rho(1-\rho) + \lambda^2\sigma^2\tau\rho^2}{(1-\lambda\iota\rho)^2},$$

where $\rho = 1 + \mu - \tau = e^{-\lambda\iota\tau}$.

4.4 The case $m_n = m$ for all n

Recall the branching process approximation result of Section 3.3, implying that the final size Z_n of the epidemic $E_{n,m}(\lambda, I)$ converges almost surely to the total progeny of a suitably chosen branching process $E_m(\lambda, I)$ as $n \to \infty$. Thus we have that

$$\lim_{t\to\infty}\lim_{n\to\infty} \mathbf{P}(Z'_n \le t) = q^m,$$

where q^m is the extinction probability of the approximating process. Choose a sequence t_n such that $t_n/n \to 0$ and $t_n/\sqrt{n} \to \infty$ as $n \to \infty$. Also, define τ as the nontrivial solution of the equation

$$1 - e^{-\lambda\iota\tau} = \tau. \tag{4.2}$$

We will show that

$$\lim_{n\to\infty} \mathbf{P}(Z'_n \le t_n) = q^m, \tag{4.3}$$

$$\lim_{c\to\infty}\lim_{n\to\infty} \mathbf{P}(t_n < Z'_n < n\tau - c\sqrt{n}) = 0, \tag{4.4}$$

$$\lim_{c\to\infty}\lim_{n\to\infty} \mathbf{P}(Z'_n > n\tau + c\sqrt{n}) = 0. \tag{4.5}$$

This means that if n is large and if the branching approximation breaks down, then the final size falls in the range $[n\tau - c\sqrt{n}, n\tau + c\sqrt{n}]$ with high probability (for some large fixed c). Scalia-Tomba (1985, 1990) has proved that the central limit theorem above (with $\mu = 0$) applies in the case of a large outbreak.

We start by proving (4.3), following Ball and Clancy (1993) rather than Scalia-Tomba (1985, 1990). Define $P_t[E_m(\lambda, I)]$ to be the probability that the branching process $E_m(\lambda, I)$ has total progeny t (including the m ancestors). If $Z'_n \le t_n$ then each infective contacts susceptible individuals at a rate bounded below by $\lambda_n = \lambda(n + m - t_n)/n$. It follows that

$$\begin{aligned}\mathbf{P}(Z'_n \le t_n) &\le \sum_{t=0}^{t_n} P_t\left[E_m\left(\lambda_n, I\right)\right] \\ &\le \sum_{t=0}^{\infty} P_t\left[E_m\left(\lambda_n, I\right)\right],\end{aligned}$$

and the right hand side is the extinction probability q_n^m of the modified branching process $E_m(\lambda_n, I)$. Now $\lambda_n \to \lambda$ as $n \to \infty$, so that $q_n \to q$. Thus, for fixed $\epsilon > 0$ there remains to choose t and n large enough that

$$q^m - \epsilon \le \mathbf{P}(Z'_n \le t) \le \mathbf{P}(Z'_n \le t_n) \le q^m + \epsilon.$$

Equation (4.3) follows. Now assume that the basic reproduction number is above 1, i.e. $R_0 = \lambda\iota > 1$, otherwise there is nothing left to prove. We proceed to show (4.4). We have

$$\mathbf{P}(t_n < Z_n' < n\tau - c\sqrt{n}) \leq \mathbf{P}(C_n(t+m) = t \text{ for some } t \in [t_n, n\tau - c\sqrt{n}])$$

$$= \mathbf{P}\left(\left[1 - e^{-\lambda\iota(t+m)/n}\right] - \frac{t}{n} = -\frac{1}{\sqrt{n}}\tilde{C}_n\left(\frac{t+m}{n}\right) \text{ for some } t \in [t_n, n\tau - c\sqrt{n}]\right).$$

Are there any values of t in the prescribed interval for which the equality above could be fulfilled? The left hand side is a concave function of t, so it is enough to check the endpoints. First put $t = n\tau - c\sqrt{n}$. After an easy calculation, we have

$$\left[1 - e^{-\lambda\iota(t+m)/n}\right] - \frac{t}{n} = \frac{c}{\sqrt{n}}\left(\lambda\iota e^{-\lambda\iota\tau} + 1\right) + O(1/n),$$

and the process $|\tilde{C}_n(t)|/\sqrt{n}$ will not be able to reach this level if c is large enough. Second, set $t = t_n$. It follows that

$$\left[1 - e^{-\lambda\iota(t+m)/n}\right] - \frac{t}{n} = (\lambda\iota - 1)\frac{t_n}{n} + O(1/n).$$

Again, this quantity is large on the $1/\sqrt{n}$ scale, since $t_n/\sqrt{n} \to \infty$ as $n \to \infty$. (Note that $\lambda\iota > 1$ by assumption.) This proves (4.4), and (4.5) is verified in the same manner.

We have thus indicated the proof of the following very important result.

Theorem 4.2 *Consider a sequence of epidemic processes $E_{n,m_n}(\lambda, I)$. Assume that $m_n = m$ for all n, and define τ as the nontrivial solution to (4.2). Also denote the final epidemic size by Z_n and write $Z_n' = Z_n + m$.*

If $\lambda\iota \leq 1$ then $Z_n \to Z$ almost surely, where $\mathbf{P}(Z < \infty) = 1$ and Z is the total progeny in a continuous time branching process $E_m(\lambda, I)$, initiated by m ancestors, in which individuals give birth at the rate λ during a lifetime distributed according to I.

If $\lambda\iota > 1$ then Z_n still converges to Z, but now $\mathbf{P}(Z < \infty) = q^m$, where q^m is the extinction probability of the branching process. With probability $1 - q^m$, the sequence $\sqrt{n}(Z_n'/n - \tau)$ converges to a normally distributed random variable with mean 0 and variance

$$\frac{\rho(1-\rho) + \lambda^2\sigma^2\tau\rho^2}{(1-\lambda\iota\rho)^2},$$

where $\rho = 1 - \tau$.

From the theorem it follows in particular that, in the case where $R_0 > 1$, the final size proportion Z_n/n converges in distribution to a random variable with mass q^m

at the point 0 and mass $1 - q^m$ at the point τ. In Figures 4.3 and 4.4 histograms of the final size in 10000 simulations are reported. Both figures treat the Markovian version of the standard epidemic model (cf. Section 2.3) and an initial population of $n = 1000$ susceptibles and $m = 1$ infectious individual. Figure 4.3 is the frequency distribution when $R_0 = 0.8 < 1$ whereas Figure 4.4 corresponds to the case where $R_0 = 1.5 > 1$. It is clear from the picture that major outbreaks occur only in the latter case. The solution of (4.2) is $\tau \approx 0.583$ when $R_0 = \lambda\iota = 1.5$ and the initial proportion infectious μ is negligible. The variance expression of Theorem 4.2 is 3.139. The theorem then states that the distribution of the major outbreak sizes should be approximately Gaussian with mean $n\tau = 583$ and standard deviation $\sqrt{3.139n} \approx 56$, agreeing quite well with the histogram.

4.5 Duration of the Markovian SIR epidemic

Let us finally discuss the *duration* T_n of the Markovian SIR epidemic, i.e. the time between the first infection and the last removal in the epidemic. Barbour (1975) has derived limit theorems, as the population size becomes large, for the distribution of the duration. The epidemic is allowed to start either with a positive fraction of infectives or with a single case. Below we give a heuristic motivation of the fact that T_n is either $O(1)$ or grows like $\log(n)$ as $n \to \infty$. We only discuss the (more complicated) case with one initially infectious individual.

Consider a sequence of standard SIR epidemics $E_{n,m_n}(\lambda, I)$, where I is exponentially distributed with rate γ. Let $X_n(t)$ and $Y_n(t)$ denote the number of susceptibles and infectives, respectively, at time t. Define the duration as

$$T_n = \inf\{t \geq 0 \,:\, Y_n(t) = 0\}.$$

We have seen (Exercise 3.3) that, if n is large, the number of infectives Y_n is well approximated at the beginning by a linear birth and death process $Y = \{Y(t), t \geq 0\}$ with birth rate λy and death rate γy. If $\lambda/\gamma \leq 1$ then this approximating process will become extinct with probability 1, corresponding to a duration T_n that is $O(1)$. On the other hand, if $\lambda/\gamma > 1$ then Y will become extinct with probability $(\lambda/\gamma)^{-1}$ and will explode with probability $1 - (\lambda/\gamma)^{-1}$. In this latter case, the approximation actually breaks down after approximately $C_1 \log(n)$ time units, as we have seen in Exercise 3.2, and we say that the *first phase* of the epidemic is over. In the *second phase* of the epidemic the bivariate process (X_n, Y_n) moves in a more or less deterministic fashion, and one can show that the duration of this deterministic phase is $O(1)$ (cf. Chapter 5). The *third phase* then begins when X_n/n has settled to $1-\tau$ but there are still infectives present in the population. Here Y_n can be approximated by another birth and death process $\tilde{Y} = \{\tilde{Y}(t), t \geq 0\}$, this time with birth rate $\lambda(1-\tau)y$ and death rate γy. We have seen in Section 4.3 that $\lambda(1-\tau)/\gamma = \lambda\iota(1-\tau) < 1$, so the approximating process $\tilde{Y}$ is always subcritical, and will therefore become extinct after an additional time $C_2 \log(n)$. Cf. the construction of Whittle (1955).

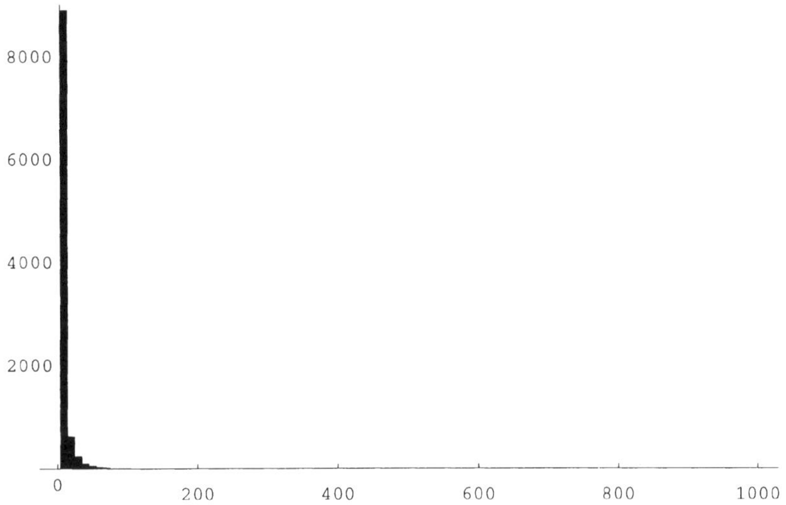

Figure 4.3: Histogram of final sizes for 10000 simulations of $E_{m,n}(\lambda, I)$ with $m = 1$, $n = 1000$ and $R_0 = \lambda\iota = 0.8$, i.e. below threshold. Each histogram bar has width 10, so for example the second bar denotes the frequency of outbreak sizes between 10 and 19.

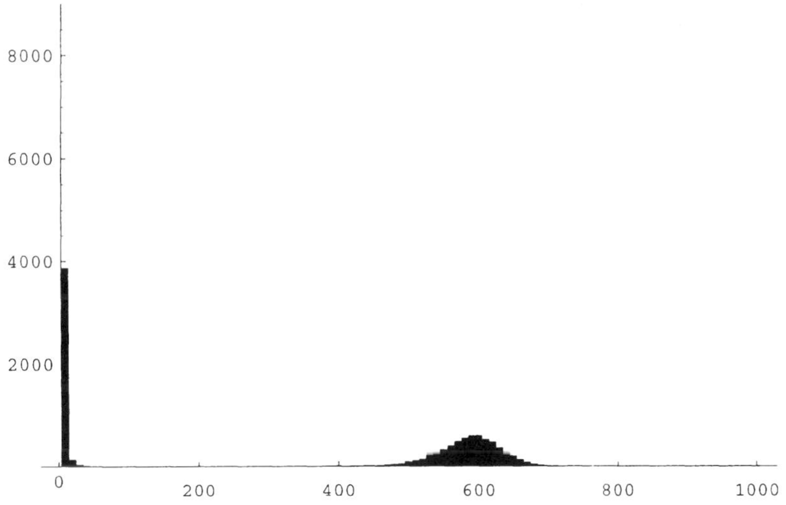

Figure 4.4: Histogram of final sizes for 10000 simulations of $E_{m,n}(\lambda, I)$ with $m = 1$, $n = 1000$ and $R_0 = \lambda\iota = 1.5$, i.e. above threshold.

These arguments together make it plausible that either T_n is short, or the ratio $T_n/\log(n)$ converges in distribution as $n \to \infty$. Actually a much stronger statement is true: Either T_n is short or the *difference* $T_n - C\log(n)$ converges in distribution as $n \to \infty$. We have the following theorem:

Theorem 4.3 *Consider a sequence of epidemic processes $E_{n,m_n}(\lambda, I)$, where I is exponential with rate γ. Assume that $m_n = 1$ for all n, and define τ as the nontrivial solution to* (4.2).

If $\lambda/\gamma \le 1$ then the duration T_n of the epidemic converges weakly to the time to extinction of a birth and death process $\{Y(t); t \ge 0\}$ with birth rate λy and death rate γy.

If $\lambda/\gamma > 1$ then the above is true only on a part of the sample space of probability mass $(\lambda/\gamma)^{-1}$. On the rest of the sample space,

$$T_n - \left(\frac{1}{\gamma - \lambda(1-\tau)} + \frac{1}{\lambda - \gamma}\right)\log(n) - c \to W,$$

in distribution as $n \to \infty$. Here $c = c(\lambda, \gamma)$ is a constant and W has the distribution of $W_1/(\gamma - \lambda(1-\tau)) + W_2/(\lambda - \gamma)$, where W_1 and W_2 are independent, both with the extreme value distribution function $F(w) = \exp(-e^{-w})$.

The proof is not difficult but rather technical, and is therefore omitted (see Barbour, 1975).

Exercises

4.1. This exercise will give you a feeling of what proportion gets infected, assuming a major outbreak, for different parameter values. Using equation (4.1), compute the (asymptotic) proportion that gets infected numerically if:

a) $R_0 = 2$ (i.e. $\lambda\iota = 2$) and $\mu = 0.1$.

b) $R_0 = 0.8$ and $\mu = 0.1$.

c) $R_0 = 2$ and $\mu = 0$ (the proportion infected is now the *largest* solution to (4.1) or equivalently (4.2)).

d) $R_0 = 0.8$ and $\mu = 0$. (What does this say about the possibility of a major outbreak?)

4.2. We know that the basic reproduction number $R_0 = \lambda\iota$ for the standard SIR epidemic remains constant as n grows. What happens with the final size if instead R_0 grows with the population size, $R_0 = R_0(n)$? Study the following cases:

a) $R_0(n) = Cn$.

b) $R_0(n) = \log(n)$.

(Hint: Since most individuals will get infected when R_0 is large, consider instead the number of individuals who *escape* the epidemic. Compute the probability that a given individual i escapes infection by looking at her threshold Q_i.)

4.3. Consider the standard SIR epidemic. Assume that $m = 1$, n is large, and the basic reproduction number is above 1. Using the branching approximation, show that the probability of a large outbreak is always less than or equal to the final size proportion in case of a large outbreak. When does equality hold? (Hint: Derive expressions for the two quantities and apply Jensen's inequality to find a relation between them.)

5 Density dependent jump Markov processes

In the present section we shall approximate certain jump Markov processes as a parameter n, interpreted as the population size, becomes large. The results will be presented in a form general enough for our purposes. More general results, as well as other extensions, may be found in Chapter 11 of Ethier and Kurtz (1986), which has served as our main source. With the aim to explain the intuition behind the theory we start with a simple example, a birth and death process with constant birth rate ('immigration') and constant individual death rate. The results in Sections 5.3 and 5.4 are applied to this example, thus giving explicit solutions. In Section 5.5 we apply the results to the Markovian version of the epidemic model described in Section 2.3. It is shown that this process converges weakly to a certain Gaussian process but in this case it is not possible to obtain explicit solutions for the deterministic limit and the covariance function. It is worth mentioning that the techniques presented in this chapter may be applied to a wide range of problems such as more general epidemic models and models for chemical reactions and population genetics, as well as other population processes.

Two fundamental results about Poisson processes will be used without proof. In Section 5.3 we use the fact that if $Y = \{Y(t); t \geq 0\}$ is a Poisson process then $\lim_{n\to\infty} \sup_{s\leq t} |n^{-1}Y(ns) - s| = 0$ almost surely, for any $t \geq 0$. In Section 5.4 we apply the result stating that the process $W^{(n)}$, defined by $W^{(n)}(t) = \sqrt{n}(n^{-1}Y(nt) - t)$, converges weakly to the standard Brownian motion. This is proven using the fact that $Y(nt) = \sum_{k=1}^{n} (Y(kt) - Y((k-1)t))$ is a sum of n independent and identically distributed Poisson random variables, and applying Donsker's theorem (e.g. Billingsley, 1968 p 68). See for example Ethier and Kurtz (1986), Exercise 4.10 for hints to a complete proof. In Section 5.4 we also integrate with respect to Gaussian processes, the so called Itô integrals. However, it is possible to read the text without any knowledge of such integrals.

5.1 An example: A simple birth and death process

Let $X = \{X(t); t \geq 0\}$ be a birth and death process with constant birth rate: $\lambda_k = \lambda$, and with death rates: $\mu_k = \mu k$. This means that individuals enter the population at constant rate λ (immigration) and each individual lives for an exponentially distributed time with mean $1/\mu$. If at time t, the process satisfies $X(t) > \lambda/\mu$, then the death rate ($=\mu X(t)$) exceeds the birth rate ($=\lambda$), and vice versa if $X(t) < \lambda/\mu$. One might therefore define λ/μ as the 'equilibrium' of the population, and one would expect the population size to fluctuate around this value, except possibly during the initial phase, if $X(0)$ is far from the equilibrium. In Figure 5.1 below a simulation of the birth and death process with $\lambda = 200$, $\mu = 1$ and $X(0) = 100$ is plotted. As we can see the process soon reaches the equilibrium value $\lambda/\mu = 200$ around which it fluctuates randomly. The arguments above are very loose, and the present chapter

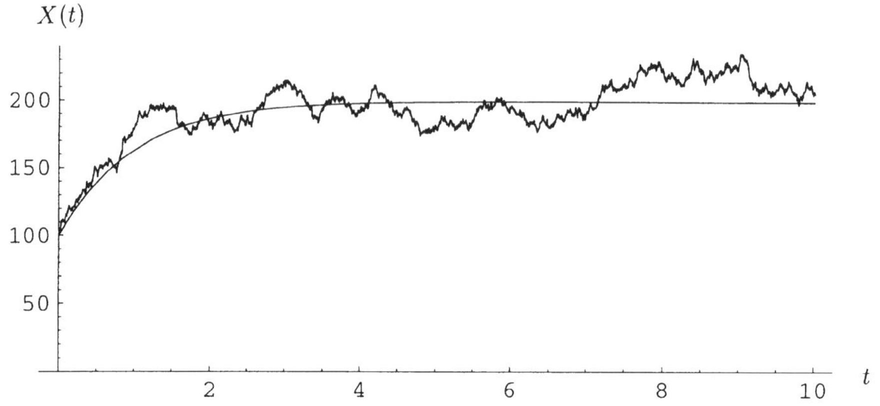

Figure 5.1: Simulation of birth and death process with $\lambda_k = 200$, $\mu_k = k$ and $X(0) = 100$.

will formalize the mathematical results. In particular, if λ is large, implying that the population size at equilibrium is large, we will show that the process above (and others of similar type) can be approximated by certain diffusion processes. For the birth and death process defined above, it turns out that it can be approximated by a so-called Ornstein-Uhlenbeck process. Such a process makes excursions away from the equilibrium, but the farther away from equilibrium the stronger is the drift towards equilibrium; a result in line with the heuristics mentioned above.

At the end of Sections 5.3 and 5.4 we apply the results of this section to the birth and death process and obtain explicit solutions. The birth and death process fits in with the model below if λ, the parameter assumed to be large, is replaced by n.

5.2 The general model

Suppose that for each $n \geq 1$, $Z_n = \{Z_n(t); t \geq 0\}$ is a continuous-time Markov process on the d-dimensional lattice $\mathcal{Z}^d$ governed by the jump intensities $q^{(n)}_{z,z+\ell} = n\beta_\ell(n^{-1}z), z, \ell \in \mathcal{Z}^d$. This means that

$$\begin{aligned} \mathbf{P}(Z_n(t+h) = z + \ell \mid Z_n(t) = z) &= hn\beta_\ell(n^{-1}z) + o(h), \quad \ell \neq \mathbf{0}, \\ \mathbf{P}(Z_n(t+h) = z \mid Z_n(t) = z) &= 1 - hn\sum_\ell \beta_\ell(n^{-1}z) + o(h). \end{aligned} \tag{5.1}$$

We assume that the process has only a finite number of possible transitions, i.e. that there are only finitely many $\ell \in \mathcal{Z}^d$ for which $\sup_x \beta_\ell(x) > 0$, and that these transition rates $\beta_\ell(x)$ are continuous functions. The starting point $Z_n(0)$ is assumed non-random. The rates above explain why the processes are called density dependent. The jump rates depend on the density of the process (i.e. normed by n). The factor

n implies that the rates increase with n, a necessary criterion for the processes to behave more and more closely like a diffusion.

One way to characterize this process is by means of Poisson processes. To this end, let $Y_\ell = \{Y_\ell(t); t \geq 0\}$ be *independent* standard Poisson process defined for each of the possible transitions ℓ. Then Z_n can be written as

$$Z_n(t) = Z_n(0) + \sum_\ell \ell Y_\ell \left(n \int_0^t \beta_\ell(n^{-1} Z_n(s)) ds \right). \tag{5.2}$$

Note that even though the Poisson processes were defined independently, the terms in the sum above are *dependent* since the observation points of the Poisson processes are dependent. It is easy to check that (5.2) satisfies (5.1) by recalling that the probability of a jump in a Poisson process in a short time interval is proportional to the length of the interval. Given $Z_n(t) = z$, the probability that there will be a jump in $Y_\ell \left(n \int_0^t \beta_\ell(n^{-1} Z_n(s)) ds \right)$ during $(t, t+h)$ is thus $hn\beta_\ell(n^{-1}z) + o(h)$, since the integrand is equal to $n\beta_\ell(n^{-1}z)$ until the first jump after t.

Note also that the processes are defined on the same probability space for different n, as the same Poisson processes are utilized in the construction. Below we prove convergence theorems for the sequence of processes $\{Z_n\}$.

5.3 The Law of Large Numbers

Before proving convergence results for $\{Z_n\}$ we derive an inequality known as Gronwall's inequality, which is interesting in its own right.

Lemma 5.1 (Gronwall's inequality). *Assume f is a real function satisfying $0 \leq f(t) \leq a + b\int_0^t f(s)ds$, for some positive constants a and b and for all $t \geq 0$. Then $f(t) \leq ae^{bt}$, $t \geq 0$.*

Proof. By iterating the inequality above one obtains

$$\begin{aligned}
f(t) &\leq a + b\int_0^t f(s_1)ds_1 \leq a + b\int_0^t \left(a + b\int_0^{s_1} f(s_2)ds_2 \right) ds_1 \\
&= a + abt + b^2 \int_0^t \int_0^{s_1} f(s_2)ds_2 ds_1 \\
&\leq a + abt + b^2 \int_0^t \int_0^{s_1} (a + b\int_0^{s_2} f(s_3)ds_3)ds_2 ds_1 \\
&= a + a(bt) + a\frac{(bt)^2}{2} + b^3 \int_0^t \int_0^{s_1} \int_0^{s_2} f(s_3)ds_3 ds_2 ds_1 \leq \ldots \leq a\sum_{k=0}^\infty \frac{(bt)^k}{k!} \\
&= ae^{bt}.
\end{aligned}$$

The result follows. •

Let $\hat{Y}_\ell$ be centered Poisson processes, that is, $\hat{Y}_\ell(t) = Y_\ell(t) - t$. Further, let $\bar{Z}_n = n^{-1}Z_n$ and define the drift function F by $F(x) = \sum_\ell \ell\beta_\ell(x)$, $x \in \mathcal{Z}^d$. With this notation, equation (5.2) is equivalent to

$$\bar{Z}_n(t) = \bar{Z}_n(0) + n^{-1}\sum_\ell \ell\hat{Y}_\ell\left(n\int_0^t \beta_\ell(\bar{Z}_n(s))ds\right) + \int_0^t F(\bar{Z}_n(s))ds. \tag{5.3}$$

The second term on the right hand side of (5.3) will be small for large n since $\sup_{s\le t} n^{-1}|\hat{Y}_\ell(ns)|$ converges to 0 almost surely, as mentioned at the beginning of the present chapter. This suggests that $\bar{Z}_n$ will resemble the deterministic vector function $z(t)$ defined as the solution to the integral equation

$$z(t) = z_0 + \int_0^t F(z(s))ds. \tag{5.4}$$

This deterministic approximation can also be explained intuitively. The process $\bar{Z}_n$ starts at $Z_n(0)$ and the 'average drift' of $\bar{Z}_n(s)$ at s is $\sum_\ell \ell\beta_\ell(\bar{Z}_n(s))ds = F(\bar{Z}_n(s))ds$, implying that $\bar{Z}_n(t)$ should be approximately equal to $Z_n(0) + \int_0^t F(\bar{Z}_n(s))ds$. The following theorem proves this strictly.

Theorem 5.2 *Suppose that* $\lim_{n\to\infty} \bar{Z}_n(0) = z_0$ *and that for each compact* $K \in \mathcal{R}^d$ *there is a constant* $M_K > 0$ *such that* $|F(x) - F(y)| \le M_K|x-y|$, $\forall x, y \in K$.

Then $\lim_{n\to\infty} \sup_{s\le t} |\bar{Z}_n(s) - z(s)| = 0$ *almost surely, where* $z(t)$ *is the unique solution to* (5.4).

Proof. The validity of the theorem relies only on β_ℓ in some neighbourhood K of $\{z(s); 0 \le s \le t\}$. Define thus $\bar{\beta}_\ell = \sup_{x\in K} \beta_\ell(x)$, which is finite due to the continuity of β_ℓ. From (5.3), the definition of $z(t)$ and the assumptions of the theorem we have

$$\begin{aligned}
|\bar{Z}_n(s) - z(s)| &= \Big|\bar{Z}_n(0) - z_0 + n^{-1}\sum_\ell \ell\hat{Y}_\ell\left(n\int_0^s \beta_\ell(\bar{Z}_n(u))du\right) \\
&\quad + \int_0^s \left(F(\bar{Z}_n(u)) - F(z(u))\right)du\Big| \\
&\le |\bar{Z}_n(0) - z_0| + \sum_\ell |\ell| \sup_{u\le s} n^{-1}|\hat{Y}_\ell(n\bar{\beta}_\ell u)| + \int_0^s M_K|\bar{Z}_n(u) - z(u)|du.
\end{aligned}$$

By Gronwall's inequality (Lemma 5.1) this implies that

$$|\bar{Z}_n(s) - z(s)| \le \left(|\bar{Z}_n(0) - z_0| + \sum_\ell |\ell| \sup_{u\le s} n^{-1}|\hat{Y}_\ell(n\bar{\beta}_\ell u)|\right) e^{M_K s}.$$

Taking the supremum then yields

$$\sup_{s\leq t}|\bar{Z}_n(s)-z(s)|\leq\left(|\bar{Z}_n(0)-z_0|+\sum_\ell|\ell|\sup_{u\leq t}n^{-1}|\hat{Y}_\ell(n\bar{\beta}_\ell u)|\right)e^{M_K t}.$$

The exponential function is independent of n, the first term in the brackets converges to 0 by assumption, and each term in the finite sum converges almost surely to 0 owing to the fact that $\sup_{s\leq t}n^{-1}\hat{Y}_\ell(ns)$ converges to 0 almost surely, for any t. This completes the proof. •

We now apply the theorem to the birth and death process defined in Section 5.1. We replace the parameter λ by n and denote the corresponding process by X_n. The two possible jumps are ± 1, and the jump rates are n for an increase and μa for a decrease if $X_n(t)=a$. With the notation of Section 5.2 this implies that $\beta_1(x)=1$ and $\beta_{-1}(x)=\mu x$. Consequently we have $F(x)=\beta_1(x)-\beta_{-1}(x)=1-\mu x$. It is easy to show that the solution to (5.4), denoted here by $x(t)$, is given by $x(t)=\mu^{-1}+(x_0-\mu^{-1})e^{-\mu t}$. By the theorem it then follows that if the initial value converges, i.e. $X_n(0)/n\to x_0$, then $X_n(t)/n$ converges to $x(t)$ almost surely, uniformly on compact sets. In particular we see that for sufficiently large t $x(t)\approx\mu^{-1}$, so $X_n(t)\approx n\mu^{-1}$, as was seen heuristically in Section 5.1.

5.4 The Central Limit Theorem

In the previous section, it was shown that the normed jump Markov vector process $\bar{Z}_n$, for a large population n, was approximately equal to the deterministic vector function z defined by equation (5.4). The next natural step is to study the deviations between the two, that is to derive a central limit theorem. As usual, it turns out that the deviations are of order $\sqrt{n}$. Before defining the $\sqrt{n}$-scaled vector process V_n we define the similarly scaled Poisson processes defined in the previous section

$$W_\ell^{(n)}(t)=\sqrt{n}\left(n^{-1}Y_\ell(nt)-t\right)=n^{-1/2}\hat{Y}(nt).$$

As pointed out at the beginning of this chapter, $W_\ell^{(n)}$ converges to the standard Brownian motion W_ℓ. The $\sqrt{n}$-scaled centered vector process V_n is then defined by

$$\begin{aligned}V_n(t) &= \sqrt{n}\left(\bar{Z}_n(t)-z(t)\right) \qquad (5.5)\\ &= v_n(0)+\sum_\ell \ell W_\ell^{(n)}\left(\int_0^t\beta_\ell(\bar{Z}_n(s))ds\right)+\int_0^t\sqrt{n}\left(F(\bar{Z}_n(s))-F(z(s))\right)ds.\end{aligned}$$

Of course, $v_n(0)=\sqrt{n}\left(\bar{Z}_n(0)-z(0)\right)$ in (5.5), which by assumption is non-random. The second equality is a direct consequence of the definition of $W_\ell^{(n)}$, $\bar{Z}_n$ and z. We can expand the integrand on the far right by Taylor's theorem, so that

$$\begin{aligned}\sqrt{n}\left(F(\bar{Z}_n(s))-F(z(s))\right) &= \sqrt{n}\partial F(z(s))(\bar{Z}_n(s)-z(s))+O(\sqrt{n}|\bar{Z}_n(s)-z(s)|^2)\\ &= \partial F(z(s))V_n(s)+O(|\bar{Z}_n(s)-z(s)|)V_n(s),\end{aligned}$$

where $\partial F = (\partial_j F_i)$ is the matrix function of partial derivatives. From Theorem 5.2 we know that $\bar{Z}_n$ converges to z, and from the beginning of this chapter that $W_\ell^{(n)}$ converges to W_ℓ, a standard Brownian motion. This suggests that V_n converges to a process V defined by the integral equation

$$V(t) = v_0 + \sum_\ell \ell W_\ell \left(\int_0^t \beta_\ell(z(s))ds \right) + \int_0^t \partial F(z(s))V(s)ds. \tag{5.6}$$

This is proven in the following theorem where we use the notation $G(x) = \sum_\ell \ell\ell^T \beta_\ell(x)$.

Theorem 5.3 *Suppose ∂F is continuous and that $\lim_{n\to\infty} v_n(0) = v_0$ (constant). Then $V_n \Rightarrow V$, the process defined in equation (5.6). This process V is a Gaussian vector process with covariance matrix*

$$\mathrm{Cov}(V(t), V(r)) = \int_0^{r\wedge t} \Phi(t,s)G(z(s))(\Phi(r,s))^T ds,$$

where Φ is a matrix function defined as the solution of

$$\Phi_2'(t,s) = -\Phi(t,s)\partial F(z(s)), \qquad \Phi(s,s) = I,$$

(Φ_2' denotes the partial derivative with respect to s).

Proof. Define $\epsilon_n(t)$ by

$$\begin{aligned} \epsilon_n(t) &= \int_0^t \sqrt{n}\left(F(\bar{Z}_n(s)) - F(z(s)) - \partial F(z(s))V_n(s)\right) ds \\ &= \int_0^t O(|\bar{Z}_n(s) - z(s)|)V_n(s)ds. \end{aligned}$$

From Theorem 5.2 we know that $\bar{Z}_n(s)$ converges to $z(s)$ uniformly on bounded intervals. Thus, since V_n is bounded in probability it follows that $\sup_{s\le t}|\epsilon_n(s)|$ converges to 0 almost surely.

Introduce $U_n(t) = \sum_\ell \ell W_\ell^{(n)} \left(\int_0^t \beta_\ell(\bar{Z}_n(s))ds \right)$ and $U(t) = \sum_\ell \ell W_\ell \left(\int_0^t \beta_\ell(z(s))ds \right)$.

These are the second terms in the defining equations of V_n and V, equations (5.5) and (5.6) respectively. Rewrite (5.5) and (5.6) to obtain

$$\tilde{U}_n(t) := U_n(t) + \epsilon_n(t) = -v_n(0) + V_n(t) - \int_0^t \partial F(z(s))V_n(s)ds. \tag{5.7}$$

$$U(t) = -v_0 + V(t) - \int_0^t \partial F(z(s))V(s)ds. \tag{5.8}$$

The processes $\{W_\ell^{(n)}; n \geq 1\}$ converge to a standard Brownian motion for each ℓ. Since $\bar{Z}_n$ converges uniformly on bounded intervals to z and ϵ_n converges to $\mathbf{0}$ it follows that $\tilde{U}_n \Rightarrow U$.

From the definition of Φ and by partial integration,

$$\begin{aligned}
\int_0^t \Phi(t,s)d\tilde{U}_n(s) &= \int_0^t \Phi(t,s)dV_n(s) - \int_0^t \Phi(t,s)\partial F(z(s))V_n(s)ds \\
&= \Phi(t,t)V_n(t) - \Phi(t,0)v_n(0) \\
&\quad - \int_0^t \left(\Phi_2'(t,s) + \Phi(t,s)\partial F(z(s))\right) V_n(s)ds \\
&= V_n(t) - \Phi(t,0)v_n(0),
\end{aligned}$$

so that

$$V_n(t) = \Phi(t,0)v_n(0) + \int_0^t \Phi(t,s)\, d\tilde{U}_n(s). \tag{5.9}$$

An identical argument shows that V satisfies

$$V(t) = \Phi(t,0)v_0 + \int_0^t \Phi(t,s)\, dU(s). \tag{5.10}$$

From equations (5.9) and (5.10) it then follows that $V_n \Rightarrow V$ by the continuous mapping theorem (e.g. Corollary 3.1.9 of Ethier and Kurtz, 1986). The vector process U is Gaussian, in fact a time-inhomogeneous Brownian motion vector. It follows that V is also Gaussian and the variance function is as specified in the theorem. •

We now apply the result to the birth and death process defined in Section 5.1. In the previous section we concluded that $X_n(t)/n$ converged to the deterministic function $x(t) = \mu^{-1} + (x_0 - \mu^{-1})e^{-\mu t}$. To simplify notation we assume that the process is started in equilibrium, that is $X_n(0) = n\mu^{-1}$ implying that $x_0 = \mu^{-1}$ and hence $x(t) = \mu^{-1}$ for all t. Since $F(x) = 1 - \mu x$ it follows that $F'(x) = -\mu$. The function Φ defined in the theorem then has the solution $\Phi(t,s) = e^{-\mu(t-s)}$, and $G(x(s)) = 1 + \mu x(s) = 2$. The theorem is applied to $V_n(t) = \sqrt{n}(n^{-1}X_n(t) - \mu^{-1})$. The assumption $X_n(0) = n/\mu$ implies that $v_n(0) = 0$ for all n, so $v_0 = 0$. The theorem then states that the scaled birth and death process V_n converges to (i.e. may be approximated by) a Gaussian process V with covariance function

$$\mathrm{Cov}(V(t),\ V(r)) = \int_0^{t\wedge r} e^{-\mu(t-s)} 2e^{-\mu(r-s)}ds = \mu^{-1}\left(e^{-\mu|t-r|} - e^{-\mu(t+r)}\right).$$

(Except at the start, i.e. for small t and r, the second term on the far right is negligible and then $\mathrm{Cov}(V(t),\ V(r)) \approx \mu^{-1}e^{-\mu|t-r|}$.) A Gaussian process having this covariance function is known as an Ornstein-Uhlenbeck process, an important process in diffusion theory (e.g. Karatzas and Shreve, 1991). It may also be illuminating to write equation (5.6) explicitly for our example:

$$V(t) = W_1(t) - W_{-1}(t) - \mu \int_0^t V(s)ds.$$

Since $W_1(t)$ and $W_{-1}(t)$ are independent their difference has the same distributional properties as $\sqrt{2}W(t)$ (where W is a standard Brownian motion, of course). Performing this substitution and writing the integral equation above as a (stochastic) differential equation we have

$$dV(t) = -\mu V(t)\, dt + \sqrt{2}dW(t),$$

which is the defining differential equation for the Ornstein-Uhlenbeck process. The properties of the birth and death process derived heuristically can be verified. The limiting process has a drift back towards equilibrium (now at the origin due to centering). Beside the negative drift, there is random noise expressed in the second term.

5.5 Applications to epidemic models

In the present section we apply the results presented above to a special case of the epidemic model defined in Chapter 2. We stress that the approximation concerns the whole epidemic process (as it evolves in time) and not only the final size as mainly studied in preceding sections. Due to the complex structure of epidemic models (although simple to define), we will not obtain very explicit solutions, as we did for the birth and death process above.

The theory involves approximations relying on the central limit theorem. This means that we can only hope to approximate the epidemic process when there are many infectious individuals, thus excluding the initial and final phases of the epidemic. We will therefore assume a (small) positive proportion of infectives when the epidemic starts; how to approximate the initial phase of the epidemic using coupling methods was described in Section 3.3. Further, we treat the special case of the standard epidemic model presented in Section 2.3 in which the infectious periods $\{I_i\}$ are exponentially distributed, making the epidemic process Markovian. By extending the dimension of the process, other distributions may be modelled using the same theory. For example, if the infectious period is $\Gamma(k, \gamma)$ the epidemic model falls under the model of Section 5.2 in which there are k infectious states, which individuals pass through sequentially with identical jump rates γ.

Using the notation of Chapter 2, the model treated in this section is denoted $E_{n,\mu n}(\lambda, I)$, where I is exponentially distributed with intensity γ. Our two-dimensional process is $Z_n = (X_n, Y_n)$, where $X_n(t)$ denotes the number of susceptibles at t and $Y_n(t)$ the number of infectives at the same time point. The initial values are $X_n(0) = n$

and $Y_n(0) = \mu n$. The proportion μ of initial infectives is assumed positive but usually very small. The process (X_n, Y_n) can make two types of jumps. Either a susceptible becomes infected, implying that the process changes by $(-1, 1)$, or else an infective is removed. The latter affects the process by $(0, -1)$. Because the infectious periods are exponentially distributed with intensity parameter γ, the jump rate for a $(0, -1)$-jump is $\gamma Y_n(t)$. New infections, or equivalently $(-1, 1)$-jumps, occur at rate $(\lambda/n) X_n(t) Y_n(t)$.

The jump intensity functions for this model are thus

$$\beta_{(-1,1)}(x, y) = \lambda xy \qquad \text{and} \qquad \beta_{(0,-1)}(x, y) = \gamma y.$$

Let $\bar{x} = x/n$, and similarly $\bar{y} = y/n$. We have then argued that the epidemic process has the following jump intensities

$$\mathbf{P}((X_n(t+h), Y_n(t+h)) = (x-1, y+1) | (X_n(t), Y_n(t)) = (x, y)) = hn\beta_{(-1,1)}(\bar{x}, \bar{y}) + o(h),$$

$$\mathbf{P}((X_n(t+h), Y_n(t+h)) = (x, y-1) | (X_n(t), Y_n(t)) = (x, y)) = hn\beta_{(0,-1)}(\bar{x}, \bar{y}) + o(h).$$

The drift function F defined in Section 5.3 is then given by

$$F(x, y) = (-\lambda xy,\ \lambda xy - \gamma y).$$

The deterministic solution $z = (x, y)$ to the integral equation (5.4) corresponds to the pair of differential equations

$$\begin{aligned} x'(t) &= -\lambda x(t) y(t), & x(0) &= 1, \\ y'(t) &= \lambda x(t) y(t) - \gamma y(t), & y(0) &= \mu. \end{aligned}$$

Recalling the historical overview in Section 1.4, we see that these differential equations are identical to those of the first deterministic epidemic model presented by Kermack and McKendrick (1927). A parametric solution to this set of differential equations was derived in Section 1.4:

$$\begin{aligned} x(t) &= e^{-\theta z(t)} \\ y(t) &= 1 + \mu - z(t) - e^{-\theta z(t)}, \end{aligned}$$

where $z(t)$ is defined by the differential equation $z'(t) = \gamma \left(1 + \mu - z(t) - e^{-\theta z(t)}\right)$, with initial value $z(0) = 0$. Here $\theta = \lambda/\gamma$.

First we apply Theorem 5.2 to show that the 'density' process $(\bar{X}_n, \bar{Y}_n) = (X_n/n, Y_n/n)$, converges to the deterministic functions defined above. To see that the conditions are fulfilled, we note that $(\bar{X}_n(0), \bar{Y}_n(0)) = (1, \mu) = (x_0, y_0)$ so the requirement that the initial value converges is obvious. Using the fact that the domain of interest satisfies $0 \leq x_1, x_2, y_1, y_2 \leq 1 + \mu$ together with the elementary bound $ab \leq (a^2 + b^2)/2$, one can show that

$$|F(x_1, y_1) - F(x_2, y_2)| \leq (2\lambda(1 + \mu) + \gamma) \, |(x_1, y_1) - (x_2, y_2)|.$$

The upper bound is just a rough estimate but sufficient for the second assumption of the theorem to be satisfied. Theorem 5.2 thus proves that $(\bar{X}_n(t), \bar{Y}_n(t))$ converges almost surely to $(x(t), y(t))$, uniformly on bounded intervals.

Theorem 5.3 can be applied to conclude that the fluctuations around the deterministic solution are asymptotically Gaussian. However, the covariance function defined in the theorem is not very explicit. Let $V_n = (\tilde{X}_n, \tilde{Y}_n)$, where $\tilde{X}_n(t) = \sqrt{n}\left(\bar{X}_n(t) - x(t)\right)$ and $\tilde{Y}_n(t) = \sqrt{n}\left(\bar{Y}_n(t) - y(t)\right)$. The matrix of partial derivatives of the drift function and the matrix function G appearing in the theorem, are

$$\partial F(x,y) = \begin{pmatrix} -\lambda y & -\lambda x \\ \lambda y & \lambda x - \gamma \end{pmatrix} \quad \text{and} \quad G(x,y) = \begin{pmatrix} \lambda xy & -\lambda xy \\ -\lambda xy & \lambda xy + \gamma y \end{pmatrix}.$$

The matrix $\partial F(x,y)$ is continuous and $(\tilde{X}_n(0), \tilde{Y}_n(0)) = (0,0)$, so the assumptions of Theorem 5.3 are satisfied. Hence, it follows that $(\tilde{X}_n, \tilde{Y}_n)$ converges to a Gaussian vector process V. The set of differential equations defining Φ in the covariance function are (derivatives below are with respect to s)

$$\begin{pmatrix} \phi'_{11}(t,s) & \phi'_{12}(t,s) \\ \phi'_{21}(t,s) & \phi'_{22}(t,s) \end{pmatrix} = - \begin{pmatrix} \phi_{11}(t,s) & \phi_{12}(t,s) \\ \phi_{21}(t,s) & \phi_{22}(t,s) \end{pmatrix} \begin{pmatrix} -\lambda y(s) & -\lambda x(s) \\ \lambda y(s) & \lambda x(s) - \gamma \end{pmatrix},$$

and with $\phi_{11}(s,s) = \phi_{22}(s,s) = 1$ and $\phi_{12}(s,s) = \phi_{21}(s,s) = 0$. It is seen that this is actually two independent pairs of differential equations. The first pair contains ϕ_{11} and ϕ_{12} and the second pair of differential equations contains ϕ_{21} and ϕ_{22} and is identical to the first one except for different initial conditions. The solutions are not explicit but can be partially derived. They are used for the computation of the covariance functions of the process, as specified in the theorem. For example, it follows from the theorem that the limit of $\tilde{X}_n(t)$ has variance

$$\int_0^t \left\{ (\phi_{11}(t,s) - \phi_{12}(t,s))^2 \lambda x(s) y(s) + \phi_{12}(t,s)^2 \gamma y(s) \right\} ds.$$

As mentioned earlier, it is complicated and not very illuminating to derive more explicit solutions. For interested readers we refer to Kurtz (1981) who characterizes the limiting process for a general distribution of the infectious period, without assuming exponentially distributed infectious periods as we have done.

Exercises

5.1. Consider the SI model (see Exercise 2.5) and assume that $m = m_n = n\mu$, so that there is a positive proportion of initial infectives. Derive a law of large numbers for $Y_n(t)$, i.e. let $n \to \infty$. (Hint: The rate of new infections is $(\lambda/n)(n + m - Y_n(t))Y_n(t)$ since there are no removed individuals and hence $X_n(t) = n + m - Y_n(t)$.)

5.2. The SI model (continued). Let $y(t)$ be the deterministic limit derived in Exercise 5.1. To simplify computations you may assume that the initial proportion infecive μ

is negligible (although positive). The central limit theorem of Section 5.4 implies that $\sqrt{n}\,(n^{-1}Y_n(t) - y(t))$ converges to a Gaussian process. Derive the integral expression of Theorem 5.3 for the covariance function. Ultimately everyone gets infected (since individuals remain infectious forever) so the variance function tends to 0 as $t = r$ gets large, but at what rate? (Hint: You may use without proof the fact that $\Phi(t,s)$ splits into a product $f(t)g(s)$.)

5.3. An SIRS epidemic is just like the SIR epidemic, only individuals in the removed state lose their immunity after some time and become susceptible again. This inflow of new susceptibles can lead to a situation where the disease 'survives' for a long time, a behaviour known as endemicity (cf. Chapter 8). . Extend the Markovian SIR epidemic to a Markovian SIRS epidemic by assuming that removed individuals become susceptible again independently at rate η. Assuming $X_n(0) = n$ and $Y_n(0) = m$ where $m = m_n = n\mu$, derive the law a large numbers for this model.

6 Multitype epidemics

The epidemic model studied so far, $E_{n,m}(\lambda, I)$, assumes that the population is homogeneous (with regard to the disease) and that individuals mix uniformly. In real life epidemics, this is rarely the case. For example, children are usually more susceptible to influenza, and sometimes individuals with a previous history of the disease have acquired some partial immunity. For STDs (sexually transmitted diseases), some individuals have higher infectivity in that they are more promiscuous (varying infectivity is often the case in other transmittable diseases as well). It may also be that the infectious periods of different individuals are not identically distributed; however, the assumption of independence seems reasonable in most cases. These heterogeneities can be characterised as *individual*. A second group of heterogeneities is caused by the social structure in the population. The model $E_{n,m}(\lambda, I)$ assumes that an individual has contact with each individual at *equal* rate ($= \lambda/n$), so that there is uniform mixing. In real life, the presence of social structures, such as households, friendly (including work) relations, and geographical structures, violates this assumption.

In the present chapter we relax these assumptions and examine the consequences to the spread of disease. In Section 6.1 we indicate how to generalise the Sellke construction and the exact results presented in Chapter 2, to the case where the contact rates between different pairs of individuals as well as the distributions of the infectious periods may vary. In Section 6.2 we discuss large population approximations. When considering a sequence of epidemic models indexed by the increasing population size, this must be done without increasing the number of parameters. We therefore treat the case where individuals in the population can be characterised by different *types* of individuals, assuming that individuals of the same type are homogeneous with respect to susceptibility, infectivity and social mixing and have the same distribution of the infectious period.

In Section 6.3 a model for epidemics among households is introduced. This model is motivated by the obvious fact that the rate of transmission tends to be much higher within households than between individuals of different households. We give some preliminary results, referring the interested reader to Ball *et al.* (1997) for the full story on household epidemics. Finally, in Section 6.4 we compare the distribution of the final size for a specific form of the multitype epidemic model with that of the final size for the 'single type' model $E_{n,m}(\lambda, I)$.

6.1 The standard SIR multitype epidemic model

The model of Chapter 2 can be generalised in a straightforward way to the case where there are different types of individuals. Before defining the model, originally considered by Ball (1986), we need some notation. Assume the population splits up into k groups of individuals labelled $1, \ldots, k$. Suppose that initially there are n_i susceptible i-individuals and m_i infectious i-individuals, $i = 1, \ldots, k$. Let $\mathbf{n} = (n_1, \ldots, n_k)$, $\mathbf{m} = (m_1, \ldots, m_k)$, $n = \sum_i n_i$ and $m = \sum_i m_i$, the latter two denoting the total number of initially susceptible and infectious individuals respectively. Finally, we let $\pi_i = n_i/n$ denote the proportion of individuals of type i (i-individuals).

Infectious periods of infectives of type i are distributed according to a random variable I_i with moment generating function ϕ_i, $i = 1, \ldots, k$, and all infectious periods are defined to be independent. Define $\iota_i = E(I_i)$ and $\sigma_i^2 = \text{Var}(I_i)$ for future use. During the infectious period of an i-individual she has contact with a given j-individual at the time points of a homogeneous Poisson process with intensity λ_{ij}/n. If the contacted individual is still susceptible, she becomes infectious and is able to infect other individuals. After the infectious period the individual becomes recovered and immune and is called removed. All Poisson processes are defined to be independent. The epidemic ceases as soon as there are no infectious individuals left in the population.

Note that λ_{ij} may not necessarily coincide with λ_{ji}. Included in this 'contact parameter' is not only the rate at which two individuals meet (naturally symmetric) but also the probability of disease-transmission which depends on the infectivity of the infective and the susceptibility of the susceptible. Some special cases of the general contact parameters $\{\lambda_{ij}\}$ have received attention in the literature. The case where the contact parameter splits up into a product $\lambda_{ij} = \alpha_i\beta_j$ goes under the name *proportionate mixing*. The parameters $\{\alpha_i\}$ and $\{\beta_j\}$ are then called infectivities and susceptibilities respectively. The case where individuals vary only in terms of their susceptibility has also received special attention. In Section 6.4, we study this case more closely and see how the heterogeneity affects the final size of the epidemic. The model defined above covers the case where all individuals are different: simply let each individual be a type of her own. The parameters of the model are the contact parameters $\Lambda = \{\lambda_{ij}\}$ and the random variables $\mathbf{I} = (I_1, \ldots, I_k)$ describing the infectious periods. Following the notation of Chapter 2 we denote the model defined above by $E_{\mathbf{n},\mathbf{m}}(\Lambda, \mathbf{I})$.

The Sellke construction can be generalised to the model above in a simple fashion. Label the i-individuals $(i, -(m_i - 1)), (i, -(m_i - 2)), \ldots, (i, n_i)$ with the infectives listed first, $i = 1, \ldots, k$. Let $I_{i,-(m_i-1)}, I_{i,-(m_i-2)}, \ldots, I_{i,n_i}$ be identically distributed random variables, each distributed according to I_i, $i = 1, \ldots, k$. Also, let $Q_{1,1}, \ldots, Q_{i,n_i}, Q_{2,1}, \ldots, Q_{k,n_k}$ be independent and identically distributed exponential random variables, having intensity 1. These are the individual thresholds. All random variables listed above are defined to be mutually independent. The initial infective labelled (i, r) remains infectious for a time $I_{i,r}$ and is then removed. Denote by $Y_i(t)$ the number of infective i-individuals at time t, and let

$$A_j(t) = \sum_{i=1}^{k} \frac{\lambda_{ij}}{n} \int_0^t Y_i(u)\, du \tag{6.1}$$

be the total infection pressure exerted on a given j-susceptible up to time t. The susceptible labelled (j,u) becomes infected when $A_j(t)$ reaches $Q_{j,u}$ and she remains infectious for a time $I_{j,u}$ and is then removed. The epidemic ceases when there are no infectives left in the population.

Exact results for the model $E_{\mathbf{n},\mathbf{m}}(\Lambda, \mathbf{I})$ are derived in a way similar to that of the homogeneous case described in Section 2.4. We shall not perform this generalisation but encourage the reader to do so. The formula for the final size can be expressed in a form similar to the final size formula for a homogeneous population. Introduce the vector notation

$$\binom{\mathbf{a}}{\mathbf{b}} = \prod_{i=1}^{k} \binom{a_i}{b_i}, \quad \text{and} \quad \sum_{\mathbf{b}=0}^{\mathbf{a}} = \sum_{b_1=0}^{a_1} \cdots \sum_{b_k=0}^{a_k},$$

and let $\mathbf{a} \le \mathbf{b}$ mean $a_i \le b_i$, $i = 1, \dots, k$. The final size of the epidemic is now specified by a vector $\mathbf{Z}$ where the component Z_i denotes the number of initially susceptible i-individuals who became infected. Let $P_{\mathbf{u}} = \mathbf{P}(\mathbf{Z} = \mathbf{u})$. Ball (1986) has shown that $P_{\mathbf{u}}$ can be derived from the recursive formula

$$\sum_{\mathbf{u}=0}^{\mathbf{v}} \binom{\mathbf{n}-\mathbf{u}}{\mathbf{v}-\mathbf{u}} P_{\mathbf{u}} \Big/ \prod_{i=1}^{k} \phi_i \left(\sum_{j=1}^{k} (n_j - v_j)\lambda_{ij}/n \right)^{u_i + m_i} = \binom{\mathbf{n}}{\mathbf{v}}, \qquad 0 \le \mathbf{v} \le \mathbf{n},$$

resembling the recursive formula for a homogeneous population in Section 2.4.

6.2 Large population limits

In the present section we discuss large population limits of the model $E_{\mathbf{n},\mathbf{m}}(\Lambda, \mathbf{I})$. We consider the case where the population size n grows but k, the number of different types, is kept fixed. A further assumption is that the matrix $\{\iota_i \lambda_{ij} \pi_j\}$, containing the expected number of contacts between all pairs of individuals, is irreducible. (A $k \times k$ matrix $A = (a_{ij})$ is called irreducible if it is impossible to find a partition $\mathcal{D}_1, \mathcal{D}_2$ of the index set $\{1, \dots, k\}$ such that $a_{ij} = 0$ whenever $i \in \mathcal{D}_1$ and $j \in \mathcal{D}_2$.) This assumption eliminates the possibility that part of the community encounters a major outbreak whereas another sub-group in the population remains unaffected. A proof of the central limit theorem for the model is very much in the same spirit as the proof for a homogeneous population in Chapter 4, but is more technical and is omitted here. A complete proof is given by Ball and Clancy (1993). Below we present and interpret the result.

Let $\pi_i^{(n)} = n_i^{(n)}/n$, $\mu_i^{(n)} = m_i^{(n)}/n_i^{(n)}$, $i = 1, \dots, k$, and assume that these quantities converge as n tends to infinity. For the limits (written without superscripts) it is assumed that each π_i is strictly positive whereas μ_i may be 0 or positive. Introduce the notation $Z_i'^{(n)} = Z_i^{(n)} + m_i$ and $\bar{Z}_i'^{(n)} = Z_i'^{(n)}/n_i$, $i = 1, \dots, k$. Thus, $\bar{Z}_i'^{(n)}$ is the proportion among the initially susceptible i-individuals who were infected during the course of the epidemic plus the ratio μ_i between the number of initially infectious and initially susceptible i-individuals. As in the homogeneous case, we distinguish between two cases depending on whether the initial number of infectious individuals is of order n (i.e. $\sum_i \mu_i > 0$) or finite.

If $\sum_i \mu_i > 0$ then the vector $\{\bar{Z}_i'^{(n)}\}$ converges in probability to τ, where $\tau = (\tau_1, \dots, \tau_k)$ is the unique solution to the equations

$$1 + \mu_j - \tau_j = e^{-\sum_i \pi_i \tau_i \iota_i \lambda_{ij}}, \qquad j = 1, \dots, k. \tag{6.2}$$

The equation above has a natural interpretation. Let $\rho_j = 1 + \mu_j - \tau_j$ be the left hand side above. Then ρ_j is the proportion of initially susceptible j-individuals who escape infection. The factor $\pi_i \tau_i$ in the exponent on the right hand side is the number of infected i-individuals (divided by n) and $\iota_i \lambda_{ij}$ is the expected infection force (multiplied by n) exerted on each j-individual. The sum in the exponent is thus the total infection force acting upon j-individuals, so the right hand side is the probability for a j-individual to escape infection. The balance equation above then simply states that the probability of escaping infection equals the proportion of individuals that escape infection. Ball and Clancy (1993) also prove a central limit theorem for the vector $\tilde{\mathbf{Z}}'^{(n)}$ with components $\tilde{Z}_i'^{(n)} = \sqrt{n_i}\left(\bar{Z}_i'^{(n)} - \tau_i\right)$. It is shown that

$$\tilde{\mathbf{Z}}'^{(n)} \xrightarrow{\mathcal{D}} N\left(\mathbf{0}, (S^T)^{-1} \Xi S^{-1}\right),$$

where S and Ξ are matrices defined by

$$\begin{aligned} S_{ij} &= \delta_{ij} - \sqrt{\pi_i \pi_j} \iota_i \rho_j \lambda_{ij}, \text{ and} \\ \Xi_{ij} &= \rho_i (1 - \rho_i) \delta_{ij} + \sqrt{\pi_i \pi_j} \rho_i \rho_j \sum_{r=1}^{k} \pi_r \tau_r \lambda_{ri} \lambda_{rj} \sigma_r^2. \end{aligned}$$

Above δ_{ij} is the Kronecker δ-function and ι_i and σ_i^2 are the mean and variance of the infectious period for i-individuals. It is worth observing that the variance increases with the variances of the infectious period, and that it coincides with the variance for a homogeneous population if there is only one type ($k = 1$).

For the second case where the number m of initially infectives is kept fixed as $n \to \infty$ Ball and Clancy (1993) prove a threshold limit theorem for the multitype model. The theorem states that $\mathbf{Z}'^{(n)}$ converges in distribution to the distribution of the total progeny of a multitype branching process having $\mathbf{m}$ ancestors, and with life distributions $\{I_i\}$ and birth rates $\{\lambda_{ij} \pi_j\}$. The basic reproduction number R_0 for the epidemic model is the largest eigenvalue of the matrix of mean offspring $\{\iota_i \lambda_{ij} \pi_j\}$. If $R_0 \le 1$ it follows from standard branching process theory (e.g. Jagers, 1975) that the total progeny of the branching process (and hence also for the epidemic) is almost surely finite. If $R_0 > 1$ there is a positive probability $1 - \prod_i q_i^{m_i}$ that the branching process explodes ($\{q_i\}$ is the solution to a certain equation). On this part of the sample space the vector $\tilde{\mathbf{Z}}^{(n)}$ converges to a normal distribution with mean $\mathbf{0}$, and the same variance as for the previous case, except for replacing each μ_i by 0 in the expression.

6.3 Household model

When modelling the spread of disease in a human population, it is very important to take into account the formation of small social groups such as households, schools and work places, the reason being that the spread of infection is usually greatly facilitated among such groups, which have a high level of mixing. Regarding household models, Ball *et al.* (1997) is the main reference. For important contributions to the theory and practical applications, see e.g. Becker and Dietz (1995), Becker and Hall (1996), Becker and Starczak (1997) and Islam *et al.* (1996). A related model is treated in an early paper by Bartoszyński (1972). Work on outbreaks within households, in the presence of community infection, but without considering the dynamics of the latter can be found in e.g. Longini and Koopman (1982), Addy *et al.* (1991) and Becker (1989). See also Andersson and Britton (1998).

Definition of the model

Initially there are n susceptible individuals and m infectious individuals. Let the susceptible population be subdivided into n/h households each of size h. (The case of unequal household sizes can be treated similarly, but the notation becomes cumbersome.) The infectious periods of different infectives are independent and identically distributed according to a random variable I. Throughout her infectious period a given infective contacts a given individual in the population (within or outside her household) at rate λ_G/n, and, additionally, a given individual in her own household at rate λ_L. If the contacted individual is still susceptible, she becomes infectious and is immediately able to infect other individuals. After the infectious period the individual becomes removed. As usual, all the random variables and Poisson processes involved are assumed to be mutually independent. Note that, by definition, infectives make both 'global' and 'local' contacts with their household members. This is for mathematical convenience only and in a large population the global rate λ_G/n can be neglected compared to the local rate λ_L.

Basic reproduction number

As usual we study a sequence of epidemic processes indexed by the population size n. The household size h is kept fixed while the number of households grows with the population size, in contrast with the situation in Section 6.1 where the number of groups was kept fixed while the group sizes grew. By using branching approximations in a heuristic way, it is possible to derive the basic reproduction number R_0. Assume that n is large and $m = 1$. The initial infective contacts on average $\lambda_{G\iota}$ individuals, and these individuals will belong to *distinct* households with high probability. Moreover, each of the individuals infected in this way generates a small sub-epidemic in her own household, comprising on average $M_L = \sum_{j=1}^{h} jP_{1j}$ individuals. Here P_{1j}, and more generally P_{ij} is defined as the probability that, given i initial infectives in the household, ultimately j household members become infected, $0 \leq i \leq j \leq h$. All these new infectives now make global contacts, introducing the disease in other households, and so on. The branching character of the number of infectious individuals is thus demonstrated, implying that the basic reproduction number R_0 is given by

$$R_0 = M_L \lambda_{G\iota}.$$

Of course, if there are no household formations ($h = 1$) we arrive at the old expression $R_0 = \lambda_{G\iota}$, whereas $R_0 = h\lambda_{G\iota}$ if the disease is highly infectious within households ($\lambda_L = \infty$).

Final size equation

Assume that n is large and that $m_n/n \to \mu > 0$ as $n \to \infty$. Let Z_n' be the ultimate number of infected individuals (including the initial infectives), and suppose that this quantity satisfies a law of large numbers, $Z_n'/n \to \tau$ in probability as $n \to \infty$. We will derive by heuristic means the asymptotic equation for τ. Define q_j to be the asymptotic proportion of households with j individuals ultimately infected, so that

$$\tau = \mu + \frac{1}{h}\sum_{j=0}^{h} jq_j. \tag{6.3}$$

Each individual in a given household of size h will become infected from outside with asymptotic probability $1 - \exp(-\lambda_{G\iota}\tau)$, and these infections occur independently of each other, thus remembering the definition of P_{ij} above it follows that

$$q_j = \sum_{i=0}^{j} \binom{h}{i} \left(e^{-\lambda_{G\iota}\tau}\right)^{h-i} \left(1 - e^{-\lambda_{G\iota}\tau}\right)^{i} P_{ij}. \tag{6.4}$$

Equations (6.3) and (6.4) together yield an implicit equation for τ. It is possible to derive rigorously the threshold limit theorem for the final size together with a normal approximation result in case of a large outbreak. The proof is very similar to the proof outlined in Chapter 4, but is notationally much more inconvenient, hence we refer to Ball *et al.* (1997) for the details.

6.4 Comparing equal and varying susceptibility

In the present section we study a specific form of the multitype epidemic model defined in Section 6.1. We assume all individuals have the same distribution of the infectious period and that the contact parameters $\{\lambda_{ij}\}$ satisfy $\lambda_{ij} = \lambda_j$. The interpretation of this is that all infectives are equally infectious – individuals only vary in terms of their susceptibility. In particular we compare the final size for such an epidemic with that of the final size of the 'corresponding' homogeneous population. In reality, one may not know which model is the correct one, thus motivating such a comparison. As a by-product we use a coupling argument to show a surprising result about exponential variables. This result was proven independently by Proschan and Sethuraman (1976) and Ball (1985). The proof below is inspired by Barbour, Lindvall and Rogers (1991). First we prove a lemma and then the main theorem concerning exponential variables, then we see what drastic consequences this has to the comparison of final size between different populations.

Lemma 6.1 *Let $\xi_1 \sim \text{Exp}(\lambda_1)$, $\xi_2 \sim \text{Exp}(\lambda_2)$ and η_1 and $\eta_2 \sim \text{Exp}(\bar\lambda)$, where $\bar\lambda = (\lambda_1+\lambda_2)/2$. Assume further that all these random variables are mutually independent. Then there exists a coupling $(\xi_1', \xi_2', \eta_1', \eta_2')$ such that $(\xi_1', \xi_2') \overset{\mathcal{D}}{=} (\xi_1, \xi_2)$, $(\eta_1', \eta_2') \overset{\mathcal{D}}{=} (\eta_1, \eta_2)$ and for which the order statistics satisfy*

$$\eta_{(1)}' \leq \xi_{(1)}', \quad \eta_{(2)}' \leq \xi_{(2)}' \qquad \textit{almost surely.}$$

In particular it follows that $\eta_{(i)} \overset{\mathcal{D}}{\leq} \xi_{(i)}$, $i = 1, 2$.

Proof. First we mention the standard way of constructing a continuous random variable X with distribution function F from a uniform random variable U. This is simply done by evaluating the inverse of the distribution function at the point U: $X = F^{-1}(U)$. It is easy to show that the random variable so obtained has distribution function F. This type of construction will be used repeatedly, without explicitly performing the transformation.

Before constructing the random variables we look at the law of the order statistics. It follows immediately from the definition of the random variables that

$$\begin{aligned} \mathbf{P}(\xi_{(1)} > t) &= \mathbf{P}(\xi_1 > t, \xi_2 > t) = e^{-\lambda_1 t} e^{-\lambda_2 t} \\ &= e^{-\bar\lambda t} e^{-\bar\lambda t} = \mathbf{P}(\eta_1 > t, \eta_2 > t) = \mathbf{P}(\eta_{(1)} > t), \end{aligned}$$

so the first order statistics are actually identically distributed. The lack of memory property for exponential variables together with the fact that η_1 and η_2 have the same intensity parameter $\bar\lambda$ implies that the conditional second order statistics satisfy $\mathbf{P}(\eta_{(2)} > t + u | \eta_{(1)} = u) = e^{-\bar\lambda t}$. In the corresponding probability for $\xi_{(2)}$ we have to condition on whichever variable is smaller. Introduce $\alpha = \lambda_1/(\lambda_1 + \lambda_2)$, so $\lambda_1 = \alpha 2\bar\lambda$ and $\lambda_2 = (1 - \alpha)2\bar\lambda$. Note that $\alpha = \mathbf{P}(\xi_1 < \xi_2)$. We then have

$$\begin{aligned} \mathbf{P}(\xi_{(2)} > t + u | \xi_{(1)} = u) &= \alpha e^{-(1-\alpha)2\bar\lambda t} + (1 - \alpha) e^{-\alpha 2\bar\lambda t} \\ \mathbf{P}(\eta_{(2)} > t + u | \eta_{(1)} = u) &= e^{-\bar\lambda t}. \end{aligned}$$

Let $f(\alpha)$ denote the right hand side of the first equation. Then $f(1/2)$ equals the right hand side of the second equation. It is easy to show that f is a convex function which attains it minimum at $\alpha = 1/2$. Hence it follows that $P(\eta_{(2)} > t + u | \eta_{(1)} = u) \le P(\xi_{(2)} > t + u | \xi_{(1)} = u)$.

Now consider the coupling. Let $U_1, \ldots, U_4$ be *i.i.d.* uniform random variables. We construct the first order statistics $\xi'_{(1)}$ and $\eta'_{(1)}$ by taking the inverse functions of U_1 (the fact that the distributions are the same implies that $\xi'_{(1)} \equiv \eta'_{(1)}$). We construct $\xi'_{(2)}$ and $\eta'_{(2)}$ using U_2 by letting $\xi'_{(2)}$ be the inverse function of the conditional distribution of $\xi'_{(2)}$ given $\xi'_{(1)}$, evaluated at U_2 and similarly for $\eta'_{(2)}$. It follows that $\eta'_{(2)} \le \xi'_{(2)}$. Finally, we use U_3 and U_4 to determine which one of ξ'_1 and ξ'_2, and η'_1 and η'_2 respectively, is the smaller. Since η'_1 and η'_2 are identically distributed, we simply let $\eta'_1 = \eta'_{(1)}$ with probability 0.5. More formally

$$\begin{aligned} \eta'_1 &= \eta'_{(1)} 1_{(U_3 \le 0.5)} + \eta'_{(2)} 1_{(U_3 > 0.5)} \\ \eta'_2 &= \eta'_{(1)} 1_{(U_3 > 0.5)} + \eta'_{(2)} 1_{(U_3 \le 0.5)}. \end{aligned}$$

We select which of ξ'_1 and ξ'_2 is to equal $\xi'_{(1)}$, so that the conditional probabilities become correct. This is done as follows

$$\begin{aligned} \xi'_1 &= \xi'_{(1)} 1_{(U_4 \le \mathbf{P}(\xi_1 \le \xi_2 | \xi_{(1)}, \xi_{(2)}))} + \xi'_{(2)} 1_{(U_4 > \mathbf{P}(\xi_1 \le \xi_2 | \xi_{(1)}, \xi_{(2)}))} \\ \xi'_2 &= \xi'_{(1)} 1_{(U_4 > \mathbf{P}(\xi_1 \le \xi_2 | \xi_{(1)}, \xi_{(2)}))} + \xi'_{(2)} 1_{(U_4 \le \mathbf{P}(\xi_1 \le \xi_2 | \xi_{(1)}, \xi_{(2)}))}. \end{aligned}$$

It is straightforward to check that this coupling satisfies the conclusions of the theorem. The distributional statement of the theorem is easy to show once the coupling has been constructed:

$$P(\eta_{(i)} > t) = P(\eta'_{(i)} > t) \le P(\xi'_{(i)} > t) = P(\xi_{(i)} > t).$$

The inequality follows trivially since $\eta'_{(i)} \le \xi'_{(i)}$ almost surely. •

The lemma above is used repeatedly in the following theorem.

Theorem 6.2 *Let $X_1, \ldots, X_n$ and $Y_1, \ldots, Y_n$ be independent exponentially distributed random variables: $X_i \sim \text{Exp}(\lambda_i)$, and $Y_i \sim \text{Exp}(\bar{\lambda})$, $i = 1, \ldots, n$, where $\bar{\lambda} = (\lambda_1 + \ldots + \lambda_n)/n$. Then there exists a coupling $(X'_1, \ldots, X'_n, Y'_1, \ldots, Y'_n)$ such that*

$$(X'_1, \ldots, X'_n) \stackrel{\mathcal{D}}{=} (X_1, \ldots, X_n) \quad \textit{and} \quad (Y'_1, \ldots, Y'_n) \stackrel{\mathcal{D}}{=} (Y_1, \ldots, Y_n)$$

and for which

$$Y'_{(j)} \le X'_{(j)}, \; j = 1, \ldots, n, \; \textit{almost surely.}$$

In particular,

$$Y_{(j)} \stackrel{\mathcal{D}}{\le} X_{(j)}, \; j = 1, \ldots, n.$$

Proof. Start with the independent sequence $X_1, \dots, X_n$. Select the first two variables X_1 and X_2 and use the lemma to construct ξ_1 and ξ_2 such that a) they are independent and both exponentially distributed with the same parameter $(\lambda_1 + \lambda_2)/2$, b) $\min(\xi_1, \xi_2) \overset{\mathcal{D}}{\leq} \min(X_1, X_2)$, and c) $\max(\xi_1, \xi_2) \overset{\mathcal{D}}{\leq} \max(X_1, X_2)$. We have thus constructed the sequence $(\xi_1, \xi_2, X_3, \dots, X_n)$ of independent exponential variables with parameters
$((\lambda_1 + \lambda_2)/2, (\lambda_1 + \lambda_2)/2, \lambda_3, \dots, \lambda_n)$ with smaller order statistics than the original sequence. The same procedure is repeated, choosing the pairs having largest and smallest λ-value, with the effect that the order statistics are reduced and the parameters are brought closer and closer to $\bar{\lambda}$. In the limit the order statistic converges to $Z_1, \dots, Z_n$ say, which has the same law as the order statistics of n independent exponential random variables with common parameter $\bar{\lambda}$. Reordering these variables at random gives a sample distributed as $Y_1, \dots, Y_n$, satisfying the statement of the theorem. The proof is complete. •

The theorem above is general and not related to epidemic models. The relevance of it for comparing the distributions of the final size for a homogeneous population with that of a population with varying susceptibility is made clear in the following corollary originally derived by Ball (1985). Below we let $(X(t), Y(t))$ denote the number of susceptibles and infectives respectively at t for the standard SIR epidemic, and $(\tilde{X}(t), \tilde{Y}(t))$ the corresponding numbers for the multitype epidemic.

Corollary 6.3 *Consider the (homogeneous) standard SIR epidemic $E_{n,m}(\lambda, I)$ and the multitype epidemic $E_{\mathbf{n},\mathbf{m}}(\Lambda, \mathbf{I})$ in which different types differ only in terms of susceptibility, and which has the same distribution of infectious periods and the same initial numbers of infectives and susceptibles as the homogeneous epidemic (i.e. all infectious periods have the same distribution as I and $\sum_i m_i = m$, $\sum_i n_i = n$ and $\lambda_{ij} = \lambda_j$). Assume further that λ and $\{\lambda_j\}$ are related by $\lambda = \sum_j n_j \lambda_j / n$. Then it is possible to construct versions $(X'(t), Y'(t))$ and $(\tilde{X}'(t), \tilde{Y}'(t))$ of the two epidemics such that*

$$X'(t) \leq \tilde{X}'(t), \text{ for all } t, \text{ almost surely.}$$

As a consequence the final sizes satisfy $Z' \geq \tilde{Z}'$ almost surely. In particular it follows that

$$X(t) \overset{\mathcal{D}}{\leq} \tilde{X}(t) \text{ and } Z \overset{\mathcal{D}}{\geq} \tilde{Z}$$

for any $n, m \geq 1$ and $t \geq 0$.

Proof. The proof follows immediately if we modify the Sellke construction slightly. Because individuals vary only in terms of susceptibility (i.e. $\lambda_{ij} = \lambda_j$) the infection pressure exerted on j-individuals, $A_j(t)$ defined in (6.1), satisfies

$$A_j(t) = (\lambda_j / n) \sum_i \int_0^t Y_i(u) du = (\lambda_j / \lambda) \tilde{A}(t),$$

where $\tilde{A}(t) = (\lambda/n)\sum_i \int_0^t Y_i(u)du$. The independent and exponentially distributed individual thresholds $\{Q_{jk}\}$ were all defined to have intensity parameter equal to 1. If we define instead the thresholds of j-individuals $(Q_{j,1}, \dots, Q_{j,n_j})$ to have parameter λ_j/λ, $j = 1, \dots, k$, then we may assume all individuals to have the same infection pressure $\tilde{A}(t)$. For this modified Sellke construction, it follows from Theorem 6.2 that we may construct individual thresholds for the two epidemics such that the order statistics for the homogeneous epidemic is smaller than those of the model with varying susceptibility. Since we may use the same realisations of i.i.d. infectious periods for both epidemics it follows that the pressure $A(t)$ for the homogeneous epidemic exceeds the pressure $\tilde{A}(t)$ in the heterogeneous model for every t using a similar argument as that used in the monotonicity result in Section 3.3. This implies that even more individuals in the homogeneous model will become infected, and so forth. •

The corollary above is not only interesting from a theoretical point of view. In real-life it is of course hard to know the susceptibilities of different individuals, even of different subgroups in the population. If all that is known is the average susceptibility the corollary then states that a homogeneous population is the worst case. That is, if we calculate the probability assuming a homogeneous population, then any heterogeneity in susceptibility can only make things better in that probability mass is shifted towards smaller outbreaks.

Andersson and Britton (1998) have argued that the calibration by comparing different models having the same *arithmetic* mean susceptibility is not necessarily a fair comparison. In fact, by the Sellke construction it seems fairer to have the same population-average of expected individual thresholds. The thresholds are exponentially distributed, so a threshold with parameter λ_i has expected value λ_i^{-1}. With this argument a population with parameters $(\lambda_1, \dots, \lambda_n)$ should be compared with a homogeneous population with parameter $\lambda_H = \left(n^{-1}\sum_i \lambda_i^{-1}\right)^{-1}$. This means that an alternative calibration is to assume that the *harmonic* means should coincide. Andersson and Britton (1998) perform this comparison and conclude that there is no corresponding strong result holding for all n and m and all t. There is one domination result stating that if m is fixed, then the *probability* of a major outbreak is minimised for the homogeneous community. Their second result holds only for the final size, assuming large outbreaks in large communities. For this case they conclude that a homogeneous population gives a larger outbreak if the disease is highly infectious, whereas some heterogeneity in the population will cause a larger outbreak if the disease is less infectious. More precisely, they show that if $\lambda_H\iota \geq 2(1-e^{-2}) \approx 2.31$ then a homogeneous model will give a larger outbreak than any heterogeneous population having the same harmonic mean susceptibility, whereas if $\lambda_H\iota < 2(1-e^{-2})$ then some heterogeneous population with the same harmonic mean susceptibility will produce a larger outbreak in case of a major outbreak.

Exercises

6.1. Consider the standard SIR multitype epidemic model with two different types and assume that the expected length of the infectious period is identical for the two types $\iota_1 = \iota_2 (=1$ say). Compute the basic reproduction number R_0 in case

a) $\lambda_{ij} = \alpha_i \beta_j$ (proportionate mixing). Extend the result to the case with k different types.

b) $\lambda_{ii} = \lambda + \delta$ and $\lambda_{ij} = \lambda$, $i \neq j$ (i.e. the mixing rate is higher within types than between).

6.2. Calculate numerically the final size vector for the two examples of Exercise 6.1 with $\pi_1 = \pi_2 = 0.5$ (in both cases), $\alpha_1 = \beta_1 = 1$, $\alpha_2 = \beta_2 = 2$, $\lambda = 1$ and $\delta = 1$.

6.3. In Section 6.4 the final size domination of a homogeneous population was established. To see if the difference is severe we here study the large population limits of the final size (Equations (4.1) and (6.2)) in some examples. Assume the initial proportion infectives is negligible ($\mu = \mu_i = 0$) and without loss of generality that $\iota = 1$.

a) Compare the final size of a homogeneous population having $\lambda = 1.5$ with the overall final size in population in which half of the community has susceptibility $\lambda_1 = 1$ and the other half $\lambda_2 = 2$ (implying the same arithmetic mean).

b) Do the same thing as in a) replacing 1.5 by 3, 1 by 0.5 and 2 by 5.5.

c) Now use the calibration suggested by Andersson and Britton (1998) to compare a homogeneous population having $\lambda = 1.5$ with a population with half of the individuals with $\lambda_1 = 1$ and the other half having $\lambda_2 = 3$ (note that the harmonic mean is unchanged).

d) Repeat c) with all parameters doubled.

7 Epidemics and graphs

Random graphs provide us with a useful tool in understanding the structure of stochastic epidemic models. By representing the individuals in a population by vertices and transmission links by arrows between these vertices, we obtain a graph that contains information on many important characteristics, such as the final epidemic size, the basic reproduction number and the probability of a large outbreak. The connection between SIR epidemics and random graphs was observed by Ludwig (1974), and has then been more fully exploited by von Bahr and Martin-Löf (1980), Ball and Barbour (1990) and Barbour and Mollison (1990). In the first two sections of this chapter the random graph interpretation of the standard SIR epidemic model will be given; we also show that the special case of a *constant* infectious period yields a particularly nice class of random graphs.

Random graphs can also serve as models of *social networks*. We can give a simple reason for introducing the network concept in epidemic modelling. Many of the classical results for the standard SIR epidemic model require the population size n to be *large*. But, according to the modelling assumptions, contacts between two given individuals in a large population occur at a very low rate; in principle, this implies that the possibility of repeated contacts is not taken into account. This observation indicates that the assumption of homogeneous mixing is not very realistic when describing epidemic spread in large populations. If we wish to allow repeated contacts between certain pairs of individuals, a possible solution is to pick a graph describing the relations between individuals, and then let the disease spread along the social network so obtained. In that way each individual is assigned to a small neighbourhood of other individuals, and can then contact each of her neighbours at a 'normal' rate. This subject is now receiving increasing attention, see e.g. Altmann (1995, 1998), Rand (1997), Diekmann *et al.* (1998) and Andersson (1998, 2000). It is far from obvious how a suitable form of the network is to be chosen. The graph should be complicated enough to catch something of the sometimes extremely irregular contact pattern in a population of living organisms, but at the same time simple enough to lend itself to mathematical analysis. Here (Section 7.3) we will just scratch the surface by explaining how to run the Markovian version of the standard SIR epidemic on a very simple network (whereby the Markov property is destroyed!).

We have so far presented various ways of modelling *social relations* in a population, ignoring completely the possibility of geographical spread of the disease. In Section 7.4 we make up for lost ground by presenting some results for a standard SIR epidemic model on the two-dimensional lattice, where the spatial element determines the progress of the epidemic completely. In order to approximate reality, social space and geographical space should of course be considered simultaneously, but to find natural models for both remains an open problem.

7.1 Random graph interpretation

Consider again the standard SIR epidemic $E_{n,m}(\lambda, I)$, endowing the individuals with random variables $I_{-(m-1)}, I_{-(m-2)}, \ldots, I_n$. Now represent the individuals by vertices of a graph, giving the vertices labels $-(m-1), -(m-2), \ldots, n$. If the ith individual ever becomes infected, we know that she will contact a given individual j in the population with probability $p_i = 1 - \exp(-\lambda I_i/n)$. Hence, for each given ordered pair (i, j) $(i \neq j)$ of vertices of the graph, let us draw an arrow from i to j with probability p_i, the presence of such an arrow having the following interpretation: "*If i ever becomes infected then i will contact j during her infectious period*". Strictly speaking, these arrows are not drawn independently, but they are conditionally independent given the I-variables. There remains only to mark the vertices $-(m-1), -(m-2), \ldots, 0$ (representing the initial infectives) and just follow the arrows. The size of the subgraph traced in this manner is exactly the final epidemic size.

The random graph obtained above can be described as a digraph (directed graph) with prescribed distribution of the out-degrees (the number of out-going arrows from a given vertex). Evidently we lose information on events referring to *time* when making this construction, since only the epidemic chain is recorded; the point is that characteristics related to the final epidemic *size* are found to have nice graph-theoretic counterparts.

As a simple application we use random graphs to indicate that even in a situation where the infectivity profile is extremely complicated, many results may be derived with the same ease as for the standard SIR epidemic. Consider the sample space consisting of all nonnegative functions $\Lambda(t)$, $t \geq 0$, with finite integral, and put some probability measure $\mathbf{P}$ on this space. Now let $\Lambda_{-(m-1)}(t), \Lambda_{-(m-2)}(t), \ldots, \Lambda_n(t)$ be an independent sample, $\Lambda_i(t)$ giving the infectiousness of individual i at time t after infection. If the ith individual ever becomes infected, she will contact a given individual j during her infectious period with probability

$$p_i = 1 - \exp\left(-\frac{1}{n}\int_0^\infty \Lambda_i(t)\,dt\right).$$

We can now draw a directed graph and trace the epidemic flow exactly as before. Using this representation, quantities such as the basic reproduction number and the distribution of the final epidemic size may easily be derived. Since latency periods and complicated time dependent infection rates can be modelled using this device, it is easy to form the impression that we have found a way to model the spread of just about any infectious disease. Note, however, that the population is still assumed to be homogeneously mixing, in the sense that all susceptibles are equally likely to contract the disease at all times; this decreases drastically the realism of the model.

Figure 7.1 illustrates such a random graph with $m = 1$ initially infectious (marked with a large black circle) and $n = 11$ initially susceptible individuals. There are

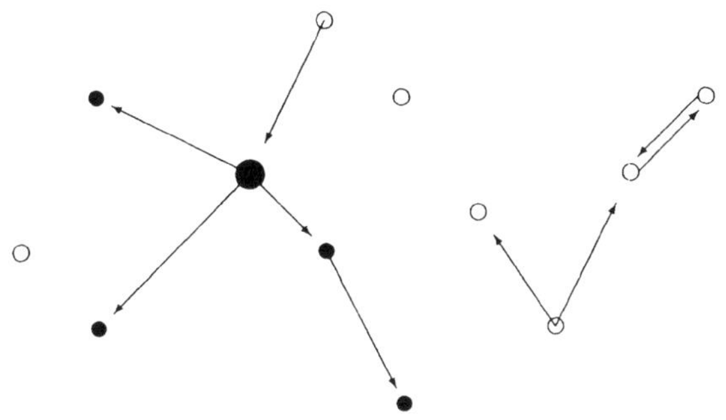

Figure 7.1: Directed graph representation of a realization of $E_{m,n}(\lambda, I)$ with $m = 1$ and $n = 11$. The initial infective is the larger black circle, while all other ultimately infected are smaller black circles. Small white circles correspond to uninfected individuals.

$Z = 4$ additionally infected in the illustration (infected individuals have smaller black circles). Note that individuals to the right do not become infected even though there are potential contacts. The reason is that the disease never reaches this subgroup. The double arrow to the far right has the interpretation that either individual could have infected the other, had she been infected.

7.2 Constant infectious period

If the infectious period in the standard SIR epidemic model is *constant*, it turns out that the random graph formulation involves the classical *Bernoulli random graphs*, which we describe next.

The theory of random graphs was introduced by Erdös and Rényi (1959) and has been extensively studied ever since. In particular, the class of Bernoulli random graphs has been very thoroughly explored, see e.g. Bollobás (1985) and Barbour *et al.* (1992). This graph model, often referred to simply as the $\mathcal{G}(N, p)$ model, is defined as follows. We are given a set of N labelled vertices. With probability p, we connect a given pair of distinct vertices i and j by drawing an (undirected) edge between them. These connections are made independently of each other. It is clear that the degree D_i of the ith vertex, i.e. the number of vertices adjacent to this vertex, is binomially distributed with parameters $N - 1$ and p, so that the average degree is given by $(N - 1)p$. In order to keep the size of the neighbourhood bounded as N grows large, we have to put $p = \beta/N$, for some $\beta > 0$. This implies that D_i will be approximately Poisson distributed with parameter β if N is large, according to the classical Poisson approximation theorem.

Two vertices i and j are said to belong to the same *component* if and only if there exists a path of edges between i and j. It is thus clear that any graph consists of a number of disjoint connected components. Properties of these components have been extensively studied for the Bernoulli graph model. In particular, the following result is well-known in random graph theory.

Theorem 7.1 *Consider the $\mathcal{G}(N,p)$ random graph model. Assume $p = p_N = \beta/N$, $N \to \infty$. If $\beta \leq 1$ then a vertex chosen at random will belong to a component of size $O(1)$. On the other hand, if $\beta > 1$ then the relative size of the largest component converges in probability to some constant C strictly between 0 and 1, as $N \to \infty$. Also, a randomly chosen vertex will belong to this giant component with probability C and it will belong to a component of size $O(1)$ with probability $1 - C$.*

Turning again to the graph interpretation of the standard SIR epidemic, let us note that if the infectious period is constant, $I \equiv \iota$, then the arrows are drawn independently of each other, and the probability of drawing an arrow from i to j is the same for all ordered pairs (i,j), $i \neq j$. Moreover, since only one (if any) of the two arrows is actually used for disease transmission, it is enough to draw one undirected edge between i and j, the presence of such an edge having the following interpretation: "If i ever becomes infected then i will contact j, and vice versa". Thus, setting $N = n + m$ and $p = 1 - \exp(-\lambda\iota/n)$, we have arrived at the $\mathcal{G}(N,p)$ random graph model!

Random graph theory can now be invoked to derive results for the corresponding epidemic process. For instance, Theorem 7.1 above immediately implies that, in the case where the basic reproduction number exceeds 1, the asymptotic probability of a large outbreak (the probability of picking a vertex belonging to the giant component) is equal to the relative size of a large outbreak (the size of the giant component). Such a result can of course also be derived by calculating the explosion probability of the approximating branching process and comparing it with the solution to the final size equation, but the graph approach gives us much more insight to the phenomenon.

7.3 Epidemics and social networks

We have indicated above how to use directed (undirected) random graphs to describe the epidemic flow, the arrows (edges) representing possible channels for disease transmission. We now proceed to show how to run an epidemic process *on* a random graph, with the edges of the graph representing relations between individuals. Individuals related in this way will be called *neighbours*. First the epidemic process on a fixed arbitrary graph is defined, and then some large population results are derived in the case where the underlying network is modelled as a Bernoulli random graph.

An epidemic process on a fixed graph

Consider a closed population consisting of $N = n + m$ individuals. Represent the neighbourhood structure in the population with a labelled undirected graph $\mathcal{G}$, so that the ith and jth vertices of the graph are connected by an edge if and only if individuals i and j are neighbours. The graph will often be the result of some random experiment. We assume that the structure is fixed during the course of the epidemic. Let G be the adjacency matrix of the graph $\mathcal{G}$, so that $G_{ij} = 1$ if i and j are connected and $G_{ij} = 0$ otherwise. It follows that G is a symmetric binary $N \times N$ matrix with zeros in the diagonal.

Let us next define the dynamics of the epidemic process. We pick m initially infectious individuals at random from the population. An infectious individual remains so for an arbitrarily distributed time period I. During this time period she makes 'close contacts' with each of her neighbours according to the points of a Poisson process with intensity λ. If the individual so contacted is still susceptible, then she will immediately become infectious. After the infectious period, the infectious individual recovers and is then immune to further infections. All infectious periods and Poisson processes are assumed to be independent of each other.

Denote the types 'susceptible' and 'infectious' by the letters X and Y, respectively. Generally speaking we set $A_i = 1$ if the ith individual is of type A, and $A_i = 0$ otherwise. Then define the number of individuals, connected pairs and connected triples with given type configurations in the following way:

$$
\begin{aligned}
[A]_n &= \sum_{i=1}^{n+m} A_i, \\
[AB]_n &= \sum_{i,j=1}^{n+m} A_i G_{ij} B_j, \\
[ABC]_n &= \sum_{\substack{i,j,k=1 \\ i \neq k}}^{n+m} A_i G_{ij} B_j G_{jk} C_k.
\end{aligned}
$$

For instance, $[XY]_n(t)$ is the number of neighbours i, j where i is susceptible and j is infectious at time t. If the total number of neighbours of a given individual is kept bounded, then all the quantities above are $O(n)$. Note that $[AB]_n = [BA]_n$, and that each pair in $[AA]_n$ is counted twice.

Bernoulli networks

As an illustration, we take the Bernoulli graph model as our underlying network. Set $N = n + m$, the total number of individuals, and put $p = \beta/n$ for some $\beta > 0$. For an outcome $\mathcal{G}$ belonging to $\mathcal{G}(N,p)$ we run an epidemic on $\mathcal{G}$, where for simplicity it is assumed that the infectious period is exponentially distributed with intensity γ.

The basic reproduction number of this model is easily derived. Introduce an infectious individual in a susceptible population consisting of n individuals, where n is large. This individual has on the average β neighbours, each of whom will become infected with probability $\lambda/(\lambda+\gamma)$, hence

$$R_0 = \frac{\beta\lambda}{\lambda+\gamma}.$$

We now describe the time dynamics of the model. Assume that the proportion m/n of initially infectious individuals tends to a nontrivial limit μ as n tends to infinity. Let us assume that $[A]_n/n$, $[AB]_n/n$ and $[ABC]_n/n$ all tend to deterministic limits as $n \to \infty$, and denote these limiting processes by a, $[ab]$ and $[abc]$, respectively. In Rand (1997) the following system of equations is derived:

$$\begin{aligned}
\frac{dx}{dt} &= -\lambda[xy], \\
\frac{dy}{dt} &= \lambda[xy] - \gamma y, \\
\frac{d[xx]}{dt} &= -2\lambda[xxy], \\
\frac{d[xy]}{dt} &= \lambda\left([xxy] - [yxy] - [xy]\right) - \gamma[xy], \\
\frac{d[yy]}{dt} &= 2\lambda\left([yxy] + [xy]\right) - 2\gamma[yy].
\end{aligned}$$

Let us explain the fourth line; the other lines are then obtained by similar reasoning. If the central individual j in a connected XXY-triple (i,j,k) is infected by the individual k, we gain an XY-pair (i,j). On the other hand, we may lose an XY-pair (j,k) in three ways: the individual j in an YXY-triple (i,j,k) is infected by the individual i; k infects j directly; k becomes removed. The fourth line now follows readily.

The system is not very useful as it stands, since no description of the time dynamics of the variables $[abc]$ is provided. Fortunately, the equations can be closed at the level of pairs by the following device. Consider a connected triple (i,j,k). Then,

$$\mathbf{P}\left(A_i B_j C_k = 1\right) = \mathbf{P}\left(A_i = 1 \mid B_j C_k = 1\right) \mathbf{P}\left(B_j C_k = 1\right).$$

If n is large, then the influence on i of the second neighbour k is negligible given the state of the first neighbour j, hence asymptotically,

$$\begin{aligned}
\mathbf{P}\left(A_i = 1 \mid B_j C_k = 1\right) &= \mathbf{P}\left(A_i = 1 \mid B_j = 1\right) \\
&= \frac{\mathbf{P}\left(A_i B_j = 1\right)}{\mathbf{P}\left(B_j = 1\right)}.
\end{aligned}$$

This translates to the formula

$$[abc] = \frac{[ab][bc]}{b} \qquad \text{for all } a, b, c.$$

Finally, we insert this relation into the system above to obtain a closed system in the five variables x, y, $[xx]$, $[xy]$ and $[yy]$. The initial conditions are given by $x(0) = 1$, $y(0) = \mu$, $[xx](0) = \beta$, $[xy](0) = \beta\mu$ and $[yy](0) = \beta\mu^2$.

This system can be simplified considerably. The equation for $[yy]$ is superfluous, since $[yy]$ does not appear in the other equations. Also the equation for $[xx]$ can be crossed out, since by writing down the differential equation for x^2 and comparing it with the differential equation for $[xx]$ it follows that $[xx] = \beta x^2$ at all times. Finally, we define $\hat{y} = [xy]/x$, the number of infectious neighbours of a typical susceptible individual. It can be verified that

$$\frac{d\hat{y}}{dt} = \frac{1}{x^2}\left(x\frac{d[xy]}{dt} - [xy]\frac{dx}{dt}\right) = (\beta\lambda x - \lambda - \gamma)\,\hat{y},$$

resulting in the differential system

$$\begin{aligned}\frac{dx}{dt} &= -\lambda x\hat{y},\\ \frac{dy}{dt} &= \lambda x\hat{y} - \gamma y,\\ \frac{d\hat{y}}{dt} &= (\beta\lambda x - \lambda - \gamma)\,\hat{y},\end{aligned} \qquad (7.1)$$

with initial condition $x(0) = 1$, $y(0) = \mu$ and $\hat{y}(0) = \beta\mu$. For a rigorous derivation of these results (and more), see Altmann (1998).

The equation for the final size proportion τ, where the proportion of initial infectives is included as in Chapter 4, is obtained as follows. Divide the third line of (7.1) by the first one and integrate to get

$$\frac{\lambda + \gamma}{\lambda}\log(x) = -\beta(1 + \mu - x) + \hat{y}.$$

At the end of the epidemic $\hat{y} = y = 0$, implying that

$$1 + \mu - \tau = \exp\left\{-\frac{\beta\lambda}{\lambda + \gamma}\tau\right\}.$$

Note that this transcendental equation is of the same form as the final size equation (4.1). The basic reproduction number R_0 appears in the formula, as it should.

It is clear that there should be a qualitative difference in behaviour between the standard SIR epidemic in a uniformly mixing population (small per capita infection rate, but a large number of individuals can be contacted) and the same type of epidemic on a social network (large per capita infection rate, but only a small number of individuals can be contacted). Indeed, an individual with an extremely long infectious period might infect a huge number of individuals under the assumption of homogeneous mixing. In a social network, however, such an individual will at most infect all of her neighbours, which is *probably* a small number, and will otherwise have no impact on the spread of the disease. Let us explore these thoughts further by indicating how to retrieve the classical Kermack-McKendrick model as a limit of (7.1) as the number of neighbours $\beta \to \infty$ and the infection rate $\lambda \to 0$ in such a way that $\beta\lambda \to b > 0$.

Using (7.1) we note that

$$\frac{d}{dt}\left(\frac{\hat{y}}{\beta} - y\right) = -\gamma\left(\frac{\hat{y}}{\beta} - y\right) + R,$$

where $R = -\lambda\hat{y}/\beta$ is small given the conditions on the parameters λ and β. Gronwall's inequality (Lemma 5.1) applied to the function $|\hat{y}/\beta - y|$ now shows that $\hat{y}/\beta$ and y coincide in the limit, hence we need not bother with the variable $\hat{y}$. We end up with the system

$$\begin{aligned}\frac{dx}{dt} &= -bxy,\\ \frac{dy}{dt} &= bxy - \gamma y,\end{aligned}$$

which we recognize as the Kermack-McKendrick model. Also, $R_0 = \beta\lambda/(\lambda+\gamma) \to b/\gamma$ which is perfectly in line with the above findings.

7.4 The two-dimensional lattice

Consider the two-dimensional lattice $\mathbf{Z}^2$. Our graph $\mathcal{G}$ is obtained by drawing an edge between two sites $i, j \in \mathbf{Z}^2$ if and only if $|i - j| = 1$ (nearest neighbour interaction). Then a Markovian epidemic process is run on $\mathcal{G}$ as described in Section 7.3 (without loss of generality, assume $\gamma = 1$). Note however that this time we are not considering a sequence of processes on larger and larger finite graphs but rather a single process on an infinite graph. This and related models have been studied in e.g. Mollison (1977), Kuulasmaa (1982), Kuulasmaa and Zachary (1984) and Cox and Durrett (1988). For an excellent introduction to the general theory of interacting particle systems and percolation processes, see Durrett (1995). Also, the book by Liggett (1985) provides a thorough treatment of the subject. Following Cox and Durrett (1988) we will discuss the critical infection rate, a quantity that corresponds to the basic reproduction number, and the asymptotic shape of the epidemic given non-extinction.

Critical infection rate

In order to discuss the critical infection rate, we again draw a directed graph to describe the disease spread without explicitly referring to the actual time dynamics. We know that a given site i will be infectious for an exponential holding time with mean 1 (if she ever becomes infected). If i contacts a given neighbour site j during the infectious period we draw an arrow from i to j, and we say in this case that the oriented bond (i, j) is *open*. Otherwise (i, j) is declared to be *closed*. Now let $\mathcal{C}$ be the set of sites that can be reached from 0 by a path of open bonds. It follows that $\mathcal{C}$ is exactly the set of sites that will ever become infected if we start by making the origin infectious. Now the critical infection rate may be defined as

$$\lambda_c = \inf\{\lambda : \mathbf{P}(|\mathcal{C}| = \infty) > 0\}. \tag{7.2}$$

By definition, a major outbreak has positive probability if and only if $R_0 > 1$. So if $0 < \lambda_c < \infty$ then our basic reproduction number may be written simply as $R_0 = \lambda/\lambda_c$, but this notation has not been acknowledged in the literature.

It is very difficult to find good bounds for the critical rate λ_c, or equivalently the critical probability $p_c = \lambda_c/(\lambda_c + 1)$. By using the so called *zero-function* and the beautiful comparison theorem of Kuulasmaa (1982) some progress can be made, as we now explain. The zero-function ϕ is defined as follows. For each subset A of $\{i \in \mathbf{Z}^2 : |i| = 1\}$ set

$$\phi(A) = \mathbf{P}(\text{all bonds } (0, i),\ i \in A, \text{ are closed}).$$

Easy calculation yields

$$\phi(A) = \frac{1-p}{1-p+p|A|}, \qquad \text{where} \qquad p = \frac{\lambda}{\lambda+1}.$$

Fix p, and consider two extreme percolation processes, with zero-functions ϕ^0 and ϕ^1 and with critical probabilities p_c^0 and p_c^1, respectively. The first one is obtained by opening the bonds with probability p independently of each other. Obviously,

$$\phi^0(A) = (1-p)^{|A|}.$$

The other extreme is obtained by, for each site i, opening *all* the bonds $(i, i + j)$, $|j| = 1$, with probability p and closing all of them with probability $1 - p$. We have

$$\phi^1(A) = 1 - p, \qquad |A| \geq 1.$$

It is easily checked that $\phi^0(A) \leq \phi(A) \leq \phi^1(A)$ for all A, and the comparison theorem tells us that $p_c^0 \leq p_c \leq p_c^1$. The number p_c^0 is exactly $\frac{1}{2}$ (see Kesten, 1982), while the other probability p_c^1 is unknown. Numerical studies in the physics literature give

$p_c^1 \approx 0.5927$. Translating to rates yields $1 \leq \lambda_c \leq 1.4552$. Simulation studies by Kuulasmaa (1982) provide us with the narrower interval

$$1.12 \leq \lambda_c \leq 1.25.$$

Asymptotic shape

Let $\zeta(t)$ be the set of removed cases at time t. If the origin is infected initially then, given non-extinction, we expect the epidemic to grow in all directions of the plane at a linear rate. The shape theorem of Cox and Durrett (1988) states the following:

If $\lambda > \lambda_c$ then, given non-extinction, there is a convex set $\mathcal{D} \subseteq \mathbf{R}^2$ such that for any $\epsilon > 0$ we have

$$t(1-\epsilon)\mathcal{D} \cap \mathcal{C} \subseteq \zeta(t) \subseteq t(1+\epsilon)\mathcal{D} \tag{7.3}$$

for t sufficiently large. Moreover, the set of infectious sites is situated close to the boundary of $t\mathcal{D}$. The set $\zeta(t)$ necessarily contains many "holes", i.e. areas of susceptible sites that are surrounded by removed sites. Not much is known about the actual shape of the set $\mathcal{D}$.

Exercises

7.1. Consider the graph interpretation of the standard SIR epidemic given in Section 7.1. Describe the distribution of the out-degrees and the distribution of the in-degrees. What happens with these distributions as $n \to \infty$, $m = 1$?

7.2. Check the details in the derivation of Eq. (7.1). Also, show that for some choices of parameter values β, λ, γ the proportion of infectives y is *increasing* initially even though R_0 is below 1.

7.3. An epidemic process on a regular network. A graph on $N = n + m$ vertices is called *k-regular* if all vertices have degree k. For N large, pick a k-regular graph at random and run the epidemic model of Section 7.3 on this graph. Assuming $m = 1$ (so $\mu = 0$ asymptotically), find conditions on (k, λ, γ) that render possible a large outbreak. Also, derive heuristically the following equation for the final size proportion τ:

$$1 - \tau = \left(\frac{\gamma}{\lambda+\gamma} + \frac{\lambda}{\lambda+\gamma}s\right)^k \quad \text{where} \quad s = \left(\frac{\gamma}{\lambda+\gamma} + \frac{\lambda}{\lambda+\gamma}s\right)^{k-1}.$$

8 Models for endemic diseases

All the epidemic models encountered so far have assumed a *closed* population, i.e. births, deaths, immigration and emigration of individuals are not considered. However, when modelling the spread of a disease with a very long infectious period or a disease in a very large population, dynamic changes in the population itself cannot be ignored. Indeed, in a large community the susceptible population might be augmented fast enough for the epidemic to be maintained for a long time without introducing new infectious individuals into the community; our common childhood diseases are typical examples. Such a disease is called *endemic*.

Already Bartlett (1956) proposed a stochastic epidemic model for endemic diseases. This model was then modified slightly into what is known as the SIR epidemic process with demography (van Herwaarden and Grasman, 1995, and Nåsell, 1999). In Section 8.1 this model is presented, and some large population results for it are given. We also discuss briefly the time to extinction of the epidemic, and the interesting notion of *critical community size*, loosely defined as the population size needed for the epidemic to persist over a given time horizon with a given probability.

Another way of achieving endemicity is to retain the assumption of a closed population, but to suppose instead that infected individuals lose their immunity after some time. It should be noted, however, that this is an artificial way to keep the epidemic going. In reality, we would not expect to observe a fixed population where individuals contract the same disease over and over again. The special case, where individuals become susceptible immediately after the infectious period, turns out to be particularly easy to analyse, much easier than the SIR epidemic with demography. This model, called the SIS epidemic model, is discussed in Section 8.2. In particular, the time to extinction is investigated in some detail. Throughout this chapter the infectious period is assumed to be exponentially distributed, thus leading to Markovian epidemic processes which can be well understood using the techniques of Chapter 5.

8.1 The SIR model with demography

Let us describe the stochastic SIR model with demography, starting with the population dynamics. Individuals are born into the population at a *constant* rate θn and each of them has an exponentially distributed lifetime with intensity θ, i.e. the average lifetime is given by $1/\theta$. The population size will thus fluctuate around the quantity n. The reason for choosing size-independent birth rates is to avoid population extinction or explosion. Assume now that the population is homogeneous and homogeneously mixing. Initially there are n susceptible and m infectious individuals in the population. A given infective stays infectious for a time period that is exponentially distributed with intensity γ (unless she dies for other causes than the disease before the end of that period). During that time she contacts a given individual at rate λ/n. If the contacted individual is susceptible, she immediately becomes infectious and proceeds to infect other individuals. All random variables and Poisson processes involved are assumed to be mutually independent.

Denote by $X(t)$ the number of susceptibles at time t, and let $Y(t)$ denote the number of infectives at time t. Then $(X, Y) = \{(X(t), Y(t)); t \geq 0\}$ is a bivariate continuous time Markov process with the following transition rates:

from	to	at rate
(i, j)	$(i+1, j)$	θn,
	$(i-1, j)$	θi,
	$(i-1, j+1)$	$\lambda ij/n$,
	$(i, j-1)$	$(\gamma+\theta)j$.

The four transitions above correspond to births of susceptibles, deaths of susceptibles, infections of susceptibles, and recovery *or* deaths of infectives, respectively. The possibility of births and deaths of individuals is the only feature that distinguishes this model from the standard Markovian SIR epidemic model. As we will see shortly, this new component in the model will have a great impact on the qualitative behaviour of the epidemic.

Law of large numbers

Consider a sequence (X_n, Y_n) of SIR models with demography, all of the processes having the same parameters θ, λ and γ. Assuming that the proportion m_n/n tends to $\mu > 0$ as $n \to \infty$, we first derive a law of large numbers for the sequence $(\bar{X}_n, \bar{Y}_n) = (X_n/n, Y_n/n)$. We wish to apply Theorem 5.2. The rates β_ℓ of Section 5.2 are as follows:

$$\beta_{(1,0)}(x, y) = \theta, \qquad \beta_{(-1,0)}(x, y) = \theta x,$$
$$\beta_{(-1,1)}(x, y) = \lambda xy, \qquad \beta_{(0,-1)}(x, y) = (\gamma+\theta)y,$$

leading to the drift function

$$F(x, y) = (-\lambda xy + \theta(1-x), \lambda xy - (\gamma+\theta)y) .$$

Exactly as in Section 5.5, we check that the conditions of Theorem 5.2 are fulfilled. Hence $(\bar{X}_n(t), \bar{Y}_n(t))$ tends to $(x(t), y(t))$ in probability uniformly on compact time intervals as $n \to \infty$, where $(x(t), y(t))$ is the solution to the system of differential equations

$$\frac{dx}{dt} = -\lambda xy + \theta(1-x),$$
$$\frac{dy}{dt} = \lambda xy - (\gamma+\theta)y,$$

with initial condition $(x(0), y(0)) = (1, \mu)$. This system cannot be solved explicitly, but we can understand its behaviour for large t by finding the stationary points, i.e. the points where the time derivatives are zero.

Let us introduce two auxiliary parameters. The basic reproduction number is given by $R_0 = \lambda/(\gamma+\theta)$, since the true infectious period is exponentially distributed with intensity $\gamma+\theta$, taking into account the possibility of death before recovery. Also, let $\alpha = (\gamma+\theta)/\theta$ be the ratio of average lifetime to average duration of infection. There are two stationary points, namely the disease-free state $(1,0)$ together with the point

$$(\hat{x}, \hat{y}) = \left(\frac{\gamma+\theta}{\lambda}, \frac{\theta}{\gamma+\theta}\left(1 - \frac{\gamma+\theta}{\lambda}\right)\right) = \left(\frac{1}{R_0}, \frac{R_0 - 1}{\alpha R_0}\right).$$

The first of the stationary points is stable for $R_0 < 1$ and unstable for $R_0 > 1$, while the second one is stable for $R_0 > 1$ (and is otherwise negative and therefore uninteresting). In other words, if $R_0 < 1$ the infection is predicted to die out fairly quickly. On the other hand, if $R_0 > 1$ then it will rise towards a positive infection level, called the *endemic level*.

Central limit theorem

Assume that $R_0 > 1$ and suppose for simplicity that the process is started close to the endemic level $(n\hat{x}, n\hat{y})$. Since the process is positively recurrent and all states (i,j) with $j \geq 1$ communicate, the process will become absorbed into the set of disease-free states $\{(i,0) : i \geq 0\}$ in finite time. Prior to absorption we expect to observe small fluctuations around the endemic level. To examine the nature of these fluctuations, define

$$\left(\tilde{X}_n(t), \tilde{Y}_n(t)\right) = \sqrt{n}\left(\bar{X}_n(t) - x(t), \bar{Y}_n(t) - y(t)\right), \qquad t \geq 0.$$

We wish to apply the central limit theorem of Section 5.4. Using the notation of that section, we have

$$\partial F(\hat{x}, \hat{y}) = \begin{pmatrix} -\lambda\hat{y} - \theta & -\lambda\hat{x} \\ \lambda\hat{y} & \lambda\hat{x} - \gamma - \theta \end{pmatrix} = \theta \begin{pmatrix} -R_0 & -\alpha \\ R_0 - 1 & 0 \end{pmatrix}$$

and

$$G(\hat{x}, \hat{y}) = \begin{pmatrix} \theta(1+\hat{x}) + \lambda\hat{x}\hat{y} & -\lambda\hat{x}\hat{y} \\ -\lambda\hat{x}\hat{y} & \lambda\hat{x}\hat{y} + (\gamma+\theta)\hat{y} \end{pmatrix} = \frac{\theta}{R_0}\begin{pmatrix} 2R_0 & -(R_0 - 1) \\ -(R_0 - 1) & 2(R_0 - 1) \end{pmatrix}.$$

Here we have expressed all quantities in terms of the new parameters R_0 and α, using that $\hat{x} = 1/R_0$, $\hat{y} = (R_0 - 1)/(\alpha R_0)$, $\lambda = \theta\alpha R_0$ and $\gamma + \theta = \theta\alpha$. It can be shown that the matrix function $\Phi(t,s)$ of Theorem 5.3 splits into a product $\tilde{\Phi}(t)\tilde{\Phi}^{-1}(s)$, hence the covariance matrix $\Sigma(t)$, $t \geq 0$, satisfies the differential equation

$$\frac{d\Sigma}{dt} = \partial F(\hat{x}, \hat{y})\Sigma + \Sigma(\partial F(\hat{x}, \hat{y}))^T + G(\hat{x}, \hat{y}), \tag{8.1}$$

by straightforward calculation using the variance expression of the theorem. We conclude that $(\tilde{X}_n, \tilde{Y}_n)$ converges weakly on compact time intervals to a Gaussian process $(\tilde{X}, \tilde{Y})$ with mean zero and covariance matrix Σ. In particular, an explicit expression for the covariance matrix for large t is easily derived as the stationary solution, $\hat{\Sigma}$, to (8.1). By easy calculation,

$$\hat{\Sigma} = \frac{1}{R_0^2}\begin{pmatrix} \alpha + R_0 & -R_0 \\ -R_0 & R_0 - 1 + R_0^2/\alpha \end{pmatrix}.$$

Time to extinction

We still assume that $R_0 > 1$. As already noted above, the time to extinction

$$T_n = \inf\{t \geq 0 : Y_n(t) = 0\}$$

from the endemic level is a.s. finite, for any fixed n. It is a classical (and very difficult) problem, going back to Bartlett (1956), to obtain estimates of this random variable. Not even the expected time to extinction is easily found. An approach that at first sight seems natural is to let the population size tend to infinity and regard disease extinction as the result of a large deviation from a high endemic level. Such an analysis is performed in van Herwaarden and Grasman (1995), who derive a complicated asymptotic formula for $E(T_n)$.

Nåsell (1999) takes a quite different approach when deriving heuristically an approximate expression for $E(T_n)$. He notes that the coefficient of variation of the number of infectious individuals in endemicity is given by

$$\frac{\sqrt{n\hat{\Sigma}_{22}}}{n\hat{y}} = \frac{\sqrt{n}\sqrt{R_0 - 1 + R_0^2/\alpha}}{R_0}\frac{\alpha R_0}{n(R_0 - 1)} \approx \frac{\alpha}{\sqrt{n}\sqrt{R_0 - 1}},$$

where the last approximation is due to the fact that $\alpha \gg R_0^2$. Indeed, if we assume that the average lifetime is 80 years and consider a disease with an infectious period of two weeks, say, then α is about 2000. Thus, even if the population size is several millions, the coefficient of variation above is still quite large. This observation suggests that for a real-life disease in a homogeneously mixing community, extinction is likely to be caused by a normal fluctuation from a not so high endemic level, rather than by a large deviation from a high level. Simulation results also show that, for realistic parameter values, the Nåsell (1999) formula gives a much better approximation to the observed time to extinction than does the formula derived by van Herwaarden and Grasman (1995).

Finally we mention the notion of *critical community size*. Needless to say, the distribution of T_n depends on the parameters R_0, α and θ as well as the population size n. The critical community size $n_c = n_c(t,p)$ with time horizon t and extinction probability p is defined as the solution n to the equation

$$\mathbf{P}(T_n > t) = 1 - p.$$

If p is small, this means that for community sizes larger than n_c the infection is likely to persist more than t time units. Nåsell (1999) obtains estimates of the critical community size for some sets of parameter values.

Below, two simulations of the SIR model with demography are shown in Figure 8.1. In both simulations $n = 100,000$, $R_0 = 10$ and $\alpha = 3750$ (corresponding to an infectious period of 1 week and average lifetime of 75 years) implying that the equilibrium is at $(n\hat{x}, n\hat{y}) = (10000, 24)$. The y-axis corresponds to the number of infectives and the x-axis to the number of susceptibles. In the top figure the disease becomes extinct rather quickly, whereas it seems to become endemic in the lower figure.

8.2 The SIS model

The stochastic SIS model for endemic infections is defined as follows. Suppose that we have a closed homogeneously mixing population consisting of n individuals. We let m of these individuals become infectious at time $t = 0$. Each infectious individual remains infectious for a time period that is exponentially distributed with parameter γ. During that time the individual makes contact with a given individual at rate λ/n. If a contacted individual is susceptible then she immediately becomes infectious. An infectious individual becomes susceptible again right after the infectious period, in contrast to the SIR epidemic models where the infectious period is followed by life-long immunity to the disease. All infectious periods and Poisson processes are assumed to be mutually independent.

Since individuals are either susceptible or infectious, it is enough to keep track of the number of individuals in the infectious state, say. Denote by $Y(t)$ the number of infectious individuals at time t. Then $Y = \{Y(t); t \geq 0\}$, can be described as a simple continuous time birth and death process on the state space $\mathcal{S}_n = \{0, \ldots, n\}$, having the following transition rates:

from	to	at rate
i	$i+1$	$\lambda i(n-i)/n$,
i	$i-1$	γi,

$Y(0) = m$. Note that we are using the *total* population size rather than just the number of initial susceptibles when scaling the infection rate. The reason is, of course, that the initial infectives may become infectious several times over the course of the epidemic and are thus taking a much more active part in the progress of the epidemic than in the SIR case, where they were merely used to start up the process.

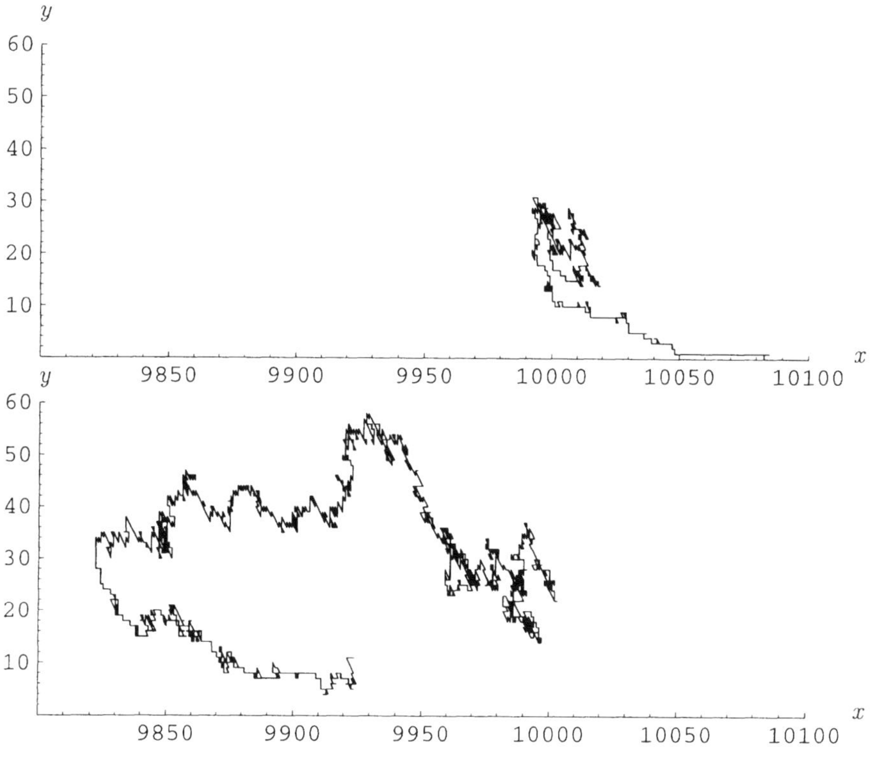

Figure 8.1: Simulations of the SIR model with demography for average population size $n = 100,000$ and equilibrium point (10000 ,24). In the top figure the disease became extinct quickly (absorbed by the x-axis) whereas the disease persisted for a long time in the bottom figure.

Law of large numbers

Consider as usual a sequence Y_n of epidemic models, all with the same infection rate λ and recovery rate γ. If the proportion of initial infectives, m_n/n, tends to a non-trivial limit μ, $0 < \mu < 1$, as n tends to infinity, we expect a law of large numbers for the scaled process $\bar{Y}_n = Y_n/n$ to be valid. To prove this, we use Theorem 5.2. Using the notation of Chapter 5, we have $\beta_1(y) = \lambda y(1-y)$ and $\beta_{-1}(y) = \gamma y$, so that the drift function is given by

$$F(y) = \lambda y(1-y) - \gamma y.$$

This function is easily seen to satisfy the condition of Theorem 5.2, hence we conclude that $|\bar{Y}_n(t) - y(t)|$ tends to zero in probability uniformly on compact time intervals as $n \to \infty$, where $y(t)$ is the solution to the differential equation

$$\frac{dy}{dt} = \lambda y(1-y) - \gamma y,$$

$y(0) = \mu$. The explicit solution is given by

$$y(t) = \frac{\left(1 - \frac{\gamma}{\lambda}\right) \mu e^{(\lambda-\gamma)t}}{1 - \frac{\gamma}{\lambda} + \mu \left(e^{(\lambda-\gamma)t} - 1\right)}$$

if $\lambda \neq \gamma$, while $y(t) = \mu/(1 + \lambda\mu t)$ if $\lambda = \gamma$. The basic reproduction number is given by λ/γ. We note that $y(t) \to 0$ as $t \to \infty$ if $\lambda/\gamma \leq 1$. On the other hand, if $\lambda/\gamma > 1$ then $y(t) \to \hat{y} = 1 - \gamma/\lambda > 0$ as $t \to \infty$. In this case, the value $n\hat{y}$ is called the endemic level of the process. Even though the deterministic motion $y(t)$ is just an approximation of $\bar{Y}_n(t)$ valid within a fixed finite time horizon, these results indicate that the stochastic SIS model will behave very differently depending on whether the basic reproduction number is below or above 1.

Central limit theorem

In order to study the fluctuations of the process Y_n, we define the $\sqrt{n}$-scaled centered process

$$\tilde{Y}_n(t) = \sqrt{n}\left(\bar{Y}_n(t) - y(t)\right), \qquad t \geq 0.$$

We restrict ourselves to the interesting case where $\lambda/\gamma > 1$ and the process is started close to the endemic level, i.e. $\bar{Y}_n(0) \to 1 - \gamma/\lambda$ in probability as $n \to \infty$. Let us apply Theorem 5.3. We have

$$\begin{aligned} \partial F(\hat{y}) &= \lambda - \gamma - 2\lambda\hat{y} = -(\lambda - \gamma), \\ G(\hat{y}) &= \lambda\hat{y}(1-\hat{y}) + \gamma\hat{y} = \frac{2\gamma}{\lambda}(\lambda - \gamma), \\ \Phi(t,s) &= e^{-(\lambda-\gamma)(t-s)}, \end{aligned}$$

and the theorem states that $\tilde{Y}_n$ converges weakly on compact time intervals to a Gaussian process $\tilde{Y}$ with mean zero and variance function

$$\begin{aligned}\operatorname{Var}(\tilde{Y}(t)) &= \frac{2\gamma}{\lambda}(\lambda-\gamma)\int_0^t e^{-2(\lambda-\gamma)(t-s)}\,ds \\ &= \frac{\gamma}{\lambda}\left(1-e^{-2(\lambda-\gamma)t}\right).\end{aligned}$$

The corresponding formulas become more complicated if the process is started away from equilibrium, or in the case where the basic reproduction number is below 1.

Time to extinction

We proceed to study the time T_n to extinction of the process Y_n,

$$T_n = \inf\{t \geq 0 \,:\, Y_n(t) = 0\}.$$

Since Y_n is irreducible on the set $\mathcal{S}_n \setminus \{0\}$ and has the state $\{0\}$ as absorbing state, the time to extinction is a.s. finite. It is of considerable interest to understand what happens to T_n as the population grows to infinity. The theorem below shows that the time to extinction for the stochastic model is a quantity that reflects the threshold behaviour of the deterministic process. In the case $\lambda \leq \gamma$ the time to extinction is always relatively short, while in the case $\lambda > \gamma$ it may be astronomical.

Before stating the result we need a definition. We say that a_n and b_n are *asymptotically equivalent* as $n \to \infty$, $a_n \sim b_n$, if the quotient a_n/b_n tends to unity as n becomes large.

Theorem 8.1 *The time T_n to extinction of the stochastic SIS model has the following asymptotic properties:*

(A1) *$\lambda > \gamma$ and $m_n/n \to \mu > 0$ as $n \to \infty$: $T_n/E(T_n) \to U$ in distribution, where U is exponentially distributed with parameter 1. Moreover,*

$$E(T_n) \sim \sqrt{\frac{2\pi}{n}}\frac{\lambda}{(\lambda-\gamma)^2}e^{nV} \tag{8.2}$$

as $n \to \infty$, where $V = \log(\lambda/\gamma) - 1 + \gamma/\lambda > 0$.

(A2) *$\lambda > \gamma$ and $m_n = m \geq 1$ for all n : $T_n \to T$ a.s. where $\mathbf{P}(T < \infty) = (\gamma/\lambda)^m < 1$. Here T is the extinction time for a linear birth and death process with birth rate λi, death rate γi and with m individuals in the beginning. On the set where T is infinite, $T_n/E(T_n) \to U$ in distribution, with U and $E(T_n)$ as above.*

(B1) *$\lambda \leq \gamma$ and $m_n/n \to \mu > 0$ as $n \to \infty$: We have that*

$$(\gamma - \lambda(1-\mu))\,T_n - \log n - \log\mu - \log\left(1 - \frac{\lambda(1-\mu)}{\gamma}\right) \to W$$

in distribution, where W has the extreme value distribution:

$$\mathbf{P}(W \leq w) = \exp\{-e^{-w}\}.$$

(B2) *$\lambda \leq \gamma$ and $m_n = m \geq 1$ for all n: $T_n \to T$ a.s. with T as in* (A2), *but now* $\mathbf{P}(T < \infty) = 1$.

The theorem states the following: (A1) If the basic reproduction number $R_0 = \lambda/\gamma$ is above 1 and the number of initial infectives is large, then the time to extinction T_n grows exponentially with the population size. (A2) If $R_0 > 1$ and we start with a small number of infectives, then a kind of threshold phenomenon presents itself. On one part of the sample space T_n stays small, on the other part T_n grows exponentially. (B1) If $R_0 \leq 1$ but the number of initial infectives is large, then T_n behaves like $\log n$. (B2) Finally, if $R_0 \leq 1$ and there is a small number of infectious individuals in the beginning then the time to extinction is always small.

Proofs and references are given in Andersson and Djehiche (1998). Below we indicate the proof of the result in the most interesting case (A2). (A1) and (A2) fall in the class of results on the exponential limiting distributions of first passage times of birth and death processes into rare sets of states, see e.g. Keilson (1979). The excellent book by Aldous (1989) gives a heuristic treatment of related topics. The results (A2) and (B2) partly rely on the coupling argument given below.

The paper by Nåsell (1996) is mainly concerned with the so-called *quasi-stationary distribution* of the process Y_n, defined by

$$Q_n(i) = \lim_{t\to\infty} \mathbf{P}\left(Y_n(t) = i \,|\, Y_n(s) \neq 0;\ 0 \leq s \leq t\right), \quad i = 1, 2, \ldots, n,$$

but interesting results concerning the time to extinction are also obtained. Nåsell notes that, for each n, T_n is exponentially distributed with parameter $\gamma Q_n(1)$ if the initial distribution of the process equals Q_n, and then uses asymptotic expansions in order to estimate $1/\gamma Q_n(1)$. In the situation (A1), and only there, whether the process is started from our prescribed fixed value or from the quasi-stationary distribution is of no importance for the asymptotic results, and indeed, in this case $1/\gamma Q_n(1)$ is asymptotically equivalent to the right hand side of (8.2). For a nice treatment of quasi-stationary distributions, see van Doorn (1991).

We now sketch a proof of (A2). By means of a simple coupling we show that, if the initial number m_n of infectives stays constant as $n \to \infty$, then the epidemic process resembles a linear birth and death process at the beginning of the time development.

Define $Z(t)$, $t \geq 0$, as a continuous time birth and death process with the following transition table:

from	to	at rate
j	$j+1$	λj,
j	$j-1$	γj,

$Z(0) = m$. It is well-known that the time to extinction T for Z satisfies $\mathbf{P}(T < \infty) = (\gamma/\lambda)^m$ if $\lambda > \gamma$. The distribution of T can be given in a closed form (see e.g. Syski, 1992). Now define a bivariate process $(\hat{Y}_n, \hat{Z}_n)$ with transition intensities

from	to	at rate
(i,j)	$(i+1, j+1)$	$\lambda i(n-i)/n$,
	$(i, j+1)$	$\lambda j - \lambda i(n-i)/n$,
	$(i-1, j-1)$	γi,
	$(i, j-1)$	$\gamma j - \gamma i$,

and initial value $(\hat{Y}_n(0), \hat{Z}_n(0)) = (m, m)$. It is clear that the marginal distributions coincide with the distributions of Y_n and Z, respectively. Moreover, $\hat{Y}_n(t) \leq \hat{Z}_n(t)$ for all $t \geq 0$. Clearly the approximation breaks down as soon as the bivariate process leaves the diagonal. By investigating the jump rates we see that downward jumps from the diagonal are impossible while upward jumps are very rare as long as the states (i,i) have $i^2 \ll n$. This implies that the two coordinates will stick together during the whole epidemic on that part of the sample space where the time to extinction of $\hat{Z}_n$ is finite. On the other hand, if $\hat{Z}_n$ explodes, then one can show that $\hat{Y}_n$ reaches the endemic level $n\hat{y}$ (or rather the integer closest to this number) with high probability.

To study the time to extinction given this latter event, we write

$$T_n = A_n + \sum_{k=1}^{K_n} B_n(k) + C_n,$$

where $A_n = \inf\{t \geq 0 : Y_n(t) = 0 \text{ or } Y_n(t) \geq n\hat{y}\}$, K_n is the number of completed excursions from the endemic level, $B_n(k)$ is the length of the kth completed excursion and C_n measures the time to reach the absorbing state counted from the time of the last entrance to the endemic level. Of course, $K_n = 0$ and $C_n = 0$ if Y_n never reaches the endemic level. By the strong Markov property, the variables $B_n(k)$ are independent and identically distributed. Also, the number of completed excursions K_n has a simple geometric distribution with parameter ζ_n, say.

The following technical results are proved in Andersson and Djehiche (1998). First, the probability ζ_n of absorption during an excursion satisfies

$$\zeta_n \sim \frac{\lambda/\gamma - 1}{2\sqrt{\lambda/\gamma}} e^{-nV} \quad \text{as } n \to \infty, \tag{8.3}$$

with $V = \log(\lambda/\gamma) - 1 + \gamma/\lambda > 0$.

Also, the expected excursion lengths satisfy

$$E(B_n(k)) \sim \sqrt{\frac{2\pi}{n}} \frac{\sqrt{\lambda/\gamma}}{2(\lambda - \gamma)} \quad \text{as } n \to \infty. \tag{8.4}$$

Finally, for any $C > 0$ we have

$$\frac{A_n}{e^{nC}} \to 0 \quad \text{and} \quad \frac{C_n}{e^{nC}} \to 0 \tag{8.5}$$

in probability as $n \to \infty$.

Using (8.5), we may write

$$\frac{T_n}{E(T_n)} \sim \frac{1}{E(K_n)E(B_n(1))} \sum_{k=1}^{K_n} B_n(k) = \frac{K_n}{E(K_n)} \frac{1}{K_n} \sum_{k=1}^{K_n} \frac{B_n(k)}{E(B_n(k))}.$$

Condition on the event that the approximating linear birth and death process explodes. Then the normed sum to the right tends to 1 in probability by a version of the law of large numbers, and it is easily checked that $K_n/E(K_n)$ tends to an exponentially distributed random variable. Also, since the expectation of T_n is asymptotically equivalent to $E(B_n(1))/\zeta_n$, Equation (8.2) follows from (8.3) and (8.4).

Exercises

8.1. Derive the differential equation (8.1) for the covariance matrix $\Sigma(t)$, $t \geq 0$, of the SIR epidemic with demography. Also derive the expression for $\hat{\Sigma}$.

8.2. Find the endemic level $(\hat{x}, \hat{y})$ for the normed SIRS epidemic $(\bar{X}_n(t), \bar{Y}_n(t))$ (see Exercise 5.3).

8.3. SIRS epidemic model (continued). Suppose that the epidemic process is started at the endemic level (i.e. $(\bar{X}_n(0), \bar{Y}_n(0)) = (\hat{x}, \hat{y})$). Apply Theorem 5.3 to derive a central limit theorem for $(\tilde{X}_n(t), \tilde{Y}_n(t)) = \sqrt{n}\left(\bar{X}_n(t) - \hat{x},\ \bar{Y}_n(t) - \hat{y}\right)$, the $\sqrt{n}$-scaled centered process.

8.4. Consider the SIS epidemic with $\lambda \leq \gamma$ and $m_n/n \to \mu > 0$ as $n \to \infty$. Give an approximation of the time until all the initial infectives have recovered from their *first* encounter with the disease, thus providing an elementary lower bound for T_n.

Part II

ESTIMATION

Until now, these lecture notes have been concerned with *modelling* the spread of disease in a community. Such modelling can be interesting in its own right and certain characteristics of the models, such as the threshold limit theorem, can provide deeper insight into the spread of disease. However, another reason for modelling epidemics is to draw conclusions about particular diseases, for the guidance of health authorities. In the sections to follow, we therefore examine the equally important area of drawing inferences about model parameters. Inference in epidemics is non-standard in that the epidemic process is often only partly observed. The available data usually consists of knowledge of those infected during the course of the epidemic, and sometimes at what time points these individuals exhibited symptoms.This implies that statistical analysis has to be based on partial observation, which, together with the strong dependencies in epidemic models, studied in Part I, makes analysis of the simplest models quite complicated.

In Chapter 9 we assume that the epidemic is observed completely, meaning that for each individual we know if she was infected or not, and if she was, the times of infection as well as removal (i.e. recovery and immunity). Such detailed data is in practice hard to collect, at least for large communities. Still, statistical methods for such data can be of interest as an indication of how much better estimates would be if such data had been available. If the answer turns out to be 'very much better' then efforts should be made to collect the necessary data.

In Chapter 10 we treat more realistic types of partial data. We concentrate on the case where the final state is observed and briefly discuss the case where the removal times of infected individuals are also observed. The statistical methods treated in Chapters 9 and 10 focus on the standard SIR epidemic model; however, methods to extend the techniques to more realistic assumptions which take account of individual heterogeneities in the community and non-uniform mixing patterns, due to the presence of social networks, are also discussed. When allowing for different heterogeneities, statistical analysis quickly becomes cumbersome, particularly in the realistic case where the epidemic is only partially observed. A different approach to statistical analysis is then to make use of Markov Chain Monte Carlo methods. This technique, which has yet to be fully developed for infectious disease data, is presented in Chapter 11.

Chapter 12 focuses on the estimation of parameters most relevant for health authorities. More important than knowing the values of certain model parameters is their interpretation in terms of how to avoid future epidemics by the introduction of preventive measures such as vaccination. More specifically, we focus on estimating the critical vaccination coverage, that is, the proportion of the susceptible population which it is necessary to vaccinate in order to prevent future outbreaks.

In Part I, we observed that if there are only few initially infectious individuals the epidemic may not take off. When drawing inferences, we can only hope for consistency in our estimation if we observe a major outbreak. Thus, one has to condition on the occurrence of a major outbreak. Rather than doing this, we take the easy way out and assume that the proportion of initially infectious individuals is positive ($\mu > 0$). In the first part of the text it was assumed that no individuals were initially immune. In reality this is rarely true: quite often there are immune individuals, possibly due to a previous outbreak of the disease. The same techniques and similar results also apply to the case with initially immune individuals, by a slight transformation of parameters. In Part II of the text we retain the assumption of no initially immune individuals. Conclusions about the parameters will be misleading if this assumption does not hold. In Exercises 9.4 and 12.2 we give hints on how to modify estimation in the case of a known positive proportion of initially immune individuals. Another problem not discussed in the text is that of model choice; we are not comparing different models statistically nor checking if data is consistent with the general model. In the present notes, parameter estimates are derived on the implicit assumption that the model is true.

We concentrate on presenting ideas and techniques for estimation, rather than actually applying the methods to real data. The main references for statistical methods for epidemics are Becker (1989) and Anderson and May (1991), with the latter excluding uncertainty considerations. The earlier monograph on modelling by Bailey (1975) also treats statistical inference. See also the recent survey paper by Becker and Britton (1999).

9 Complete observation of the epidemic process

In this chapter we assume that the standard SIR epidemic process $E_{n,m}(\lambda, I)$ is observed completely. By complete observation is meant that the infection times τ_i and removal times ρ_i (hence also the length of the infectious period $I_i = \rho_i - \tau_i$) of all infected individuals are observed; for individuals who did not become infected we define $\tau_i = \infty$ and $I_i = 0$ for formulas to be consistent. From the data it is obviously possible to deduce how many individuals are susceptible, infectious (and removed) for each time t, implying that $(X, Y) = \{(X(t), Y(t)); t \geq 0\}$ as well as the final size $Z = n - X(\infty)$ are observed. Based on the observed data we want to draw inferences on the transmission parameter λ and the distribution of the infectious period I. We do this by means of Maximum Likelihood (ML) theory. First, we have to make the meaning of 'likelihood' clear for such epidemic processes. Hence, in Section 9.1 we derive the log-likelihood for a vector of counting processes, and also state some properties of martingales which will turn out useful in the statistical analysis.

9.1 Martingales and log-likelihoods of counting processes

An excellent reference to statistical methods for counting process data is Andersen *et al.* (1993), where both theory and many examples are given. In the present section we state some results and motivate them heuristically. Consider a vector of counting processes $N = (N_1, \ldots, N_k)$, where each component $N_i(t)$ counts the *number* of times a specific event has occurred up to time t. Assume that the probability that such an event occurs in $(t, t+h]$ given the history of the whole vector process up until t, denoted $\mathcal{H}_t$, satisfies

$$\begin{aligned} \mathbf{P}(N_i(t+h) - N_i(t) = 1 \mid \mathcal{H}_t) &= h\lambda_i(t) + o(h), \quad i = 1, \ldots, k, \\ \mathbf{P}(N(t+h) - N(t) = 0 \mid \mathcal{H}_t) &= 1 - h\sum_i \lambda_i(t) + o(h). \end{aligned} \tag{9.1}$$

In the equations above $\lambda_i(t)$, denoted intensity functions, are non-negative functions which may depend on the history of the process up until time t. Formally this is written as $\lambda_i(t) \in \mathcal{H}_t$ and $(\mathcal{H}_t)_{t\geq 0}$ is called a filtration of σ-fields. To go into mathematical details is beyond the scope of these lecture notes – often, it suffices to understand their meaning heuristically. The equations above imply that, in a short time interval, only one of the k different events can occur (i.e. the corresponding counting process increases by 1). Notice the similarities between (9.1) and the jump rates (5.1) of Chapter 5. The intensities above are more general in that they may also depend on the process prior to t (i.e. the process is not necessarily Markovian), and less general in that only one type of jump (increase by 1) can occur.

What is the log-likelihood of the observations on $\{N(t); 0 \leq t \leq u)\}$ for this process? We derive this heuristically by dividing $(0, u)$ into small increments Δ_t of length h and working out the probability of observing what happens in the increment, conditional on the history prior to the increment. Let $\Delta_t = [t, t+h)$ and let $\Delta N_i(t) = N_i(t+h) - N_i(t)$ be the number of i-events that occur in this interval. Then the probability of our observations can be written as

$$\prod_{\Delta_t \subset (0,u)} \left(\prod_i \left((h\lambda_i(t))^{\Delta N_i(t)} \right) \left(1 - h \sum_i \lambda_i(t) \right)^{1-\sum_i \Delta N_i(t)} + o(h) \right).$$

The two factors within the large brackets above simply pick out which of the probabilities to use, depending on what was observed in Δ_t. As the increment length h becomes smaller, the number of increments increases and all but the increments containing events appear in the second factor above. For small h this factor is equivalent to $\exp\left(-h \sum_i \lambda_i(t)\right)$. The expression above decreases (except if no events have occurred) because of the h's appearing in the inner product. This is not surprising: the probability of observing the events *exactly* at some given time points is 0! However, if we divide the expression above by h to a power equal to the observed number of jumps, and let h tend to 0, it can be shown that the *logarithm* of the expression above converges to

$$\ell_u(N(t); 0 \le t \le u) = \sum_i \int_0^u (\log[\lambda_i(t-)]dN_i(t) - \lambda_i(t-)dt), \tag{9.2}$$

and this is the log-likelihood of the observed process, with $\lambda_i(t-)$ denoting the intensity just before t. In the expression above $dN_i(t)$ is 1 at times t when the counting process increases, and 0 otherwise, so the first integral is actually a sum.

The log-likelihood is used for drawing inferences about parameter(s) θ of the intensity functions. From now on, we therefore write $\lambda_i(\theta; t-)$ and $\ell_u(\theta)$ for the intensities and the log-likelihood respectively. Below a one dimensional parameter is considered, otherwise partial derivatives should be used. The true, unknown parameter value is denoted by θ_0. Further, all derivatives will be with respect to the parameter and not time. If we have observed the counting process up until u, the ML-estimator $\hat{\theta}_u$ is the solution θ which maximizes $\ell_u(\theta)$. We find the maximum by differentiating the log-likelihood:

$$\begin{aligned} \ell_u'(\theta) &= \sum_i \int_0^u \left(\frac{\lambda_i'(\theta; t-)}{\lambda_i(\theta; t-)} dN_i(t) - \lambda_i'(\theta, t-)dt\right) \\ &= \sum_i \int_0^u \frac{\lambda_i'(\theta; t-)}{\lambda_i(\theta; t-)} (dN_i(t) - \lambda_i(\theta, t-)dt). \end{aligned} \tag{9.3}$$

The process above, viewed as a function of u is often called the score process in statistical literature. The ML-estimator $\hat{\theta}$ is the solution of the equation $\ell_u'(\theta) = 0$.

For the true parameter θ_0, i.e. using the true intensities, the integration increments $dN_i(t) - \lambda_i(\theta_0, t-)dt$ have zero mean (cf. Equation 9.1). Such zero-mean increments are closely connected to martingales, a notion we now describe.

A process $M = \{M_u; u \geq 0\}$ is said to be a martingale (with respect to the history $\mathcal{H}_t$) if it satisfies two conditions: $E(|M_u|) < \infty$ for all u, and $E(M_u|\mathcal{H}_t) = M_t$ for $u \geq t$. The theory of martingales is rich and profound; a rigorous presentation is given in Andersen *et al.* (1993), Chapter II, and a less mathematical description with a view to applications in epidemics is to be found in Becker (1989), Chapter 7. We now state some properties of martingales relevant for our application (here we only consider 1-dimensional martingales, but many results can be extended to the multivariate case). The single most important property of a martingale M is the second defining property, namely that its expected future value equals its present value. In our case the martingale will be $\ell_u(\theta_0)$ which is 0 at $u = 0$, implying that $E(\ell_u(\theta_0)) = 0$ for all u. Further, a linear combination $aM + b\tilde{M}$ of martingales is a martingale. If a bounded predictable process, i.e. a bounded process X for which X(t) is determined by $\mathcal{H}_{t-}$ (the history up to but not including t), is integrated with respect to a martingale M, then the resulting process $\tilde{M}(t) = \int_0^t X(u)dM(u)$ is a martingale.

From the properties stated above it follows that the score process $\{\ell_u(\theta_0); u \geq 0\}$, evaluated at the true parameter value θ_0, is a martingale. For many martingales it is possible to prove central limit theorems as some quantity tends to infinity. In addition to the mean we therefore need to derive the variance of a martingale. Consider a martingale of the form $M_u = \int_0^u f(t)(dN(t) - \lambda(t-)dt)$, where $N(t)$ is a counting process with intensity $\lambda(t)$ and f is a predictable process (as in our case above). Define the so-called optional and predictable variation processes by $[M]_u = \int_0^u f^2(t)dN(t)$ and $\langle M\rangle_u = \int_0^u f^2(t)\lambda(t-)dt$ respectively. The following lemma explains why they are called variation processes.

Lemma 9.1 *Suppose the martingale M defined above has finite second order moments. Then* $\text{Var}(M_u) = E[\langle M\rangle_u] = E[[M]_u]$.

Proof. The second equality is immediate since $[M]_u - \langle M\rangle_u = \int_0^\infty f^2(t)(dN(t) - \lambda(t-)dt)$ is itself a martingale, so its expectation is 0. The first equality is derived as follows. The defining integral of M_u is the limit of the sum $\sum_{\Delta_t} f(t)(\Delta N(t) - \lambda(t)h)$ using the same notation as before. The variance of such a sum is the sum of covariances. Each such covariance term is equal to the expectation of the product since

$$
\begin{aligned}
E[f(t)(\Delta N(t) - \lambda(t)h)] &= E[E[f(t)(\Delta N(t) - \lambda(t)h)|\mathcal{H}_t]] \\
&= E[f(t)E[\Delta N(t) - \lambda(t)h|\mathcal{H}_t]] \\
&= 0.
\end{aligned}
$$

This follows because the increments have mean 0. Consider a covariance term with disjoint time intervals Δ_s and Δ_t where $s+h<t$. Then

$$\begin{aligned}
&E[f(s)(\Delta N(s)-\lambda(s)h)f(t)(\Delta N(t)-\lambda(t)h)]\\
&=E[E[f(s)(\Delta N(s)-\lambda(s)h)f(t)(\Delta N(t)-\lambda(t)h)|\mathcal{H}_{s+h}]]\\
&=E[f(s)(\Delta N(s)-\lambda(s)h)E[f(t)(\Delta N(t)-\lambda(t)h)|\mathcal{H}_{s+h}]]\\
&=0.
\end{aligned}$$

The covariance between terms of disjoint time intervals is hence 0. Now the diagonal terms, i.e. the variance terms, are

$$\mathrm{Var}[f(t)(\Delta N(t)-\lambda(t)h)]=E[f^2(t)(\Delta N(t)-\lambda(t)h)^2]=E[f^2(t)E[(\Delta N(t)-\lambda(t)h)^2|\mathcal{H}_t]].$$

The factor inside the inner expectation takes the value $(-\lambda(t)h)^2$ if there is no jump in the interval and the value $(1-\lambda(t)h)^2\approx 1$ if there is a jump, and the latter happens with probability $\lambda(t)h$. Neglecting terms of order $o(h)$ we thus have $E[(\Delta N(t)-\lambda(t)h)^2|\mathcal{H}_{t-}]=\lambda(t)h$ and consequently the variance term equals $E[f^2(t)\lambda(t)h]$. The variance of the sum hence equals the sum of variances:

$$\mathrm{Var}[M_u]=\sum_{\Delta_t}E[f^2(t)\lambda(t)h+o(h)]=E[\sum_{\Delta_t}f^2(t)\lambda(t)h+o(h)].$$

Taking smaller and smaller intervals shows that this converges to $E[\int_0^u f^2(t)\lambda(t-)dt]$ as stated. •

Using the same technique one can prove the following lemma stating that martingales from counting processes with no simultaneous jumps are uncorrelated.

Lemma 9.2 *Consider two martingales M_1 and M_2 defined by*

$$\begin{aligned}
M_1(u) &= \int_0^u f_1(t)(dN_1(t)-\lambda_1(t-)dt),\\
M_2(u) &= \int_0^u f_2(t)(dN_2(t)-\lambda_2(t-)dt),
\end{aligned}$$

where N_1 and N_2 are counting processes without simultaneous jumps having intensities λ_1 and λ_2 respectively and f_1 and f_2 are predictable processes. Then the covariance function satisfies $\mathrm{Cov}(M_1(u),\ M_2(t))=0$ *for all* $u,\ t\geq 0$.

Proof. The lemma is proven using methods similar to those in the proof of Lemma 9.1. Hints are given in Exercise 9.1. •

We conclude this section by stating a martingale central limit theorem due to Rebolledo (1980) (see also Andersen *et al.*, 1993, p 83). For this we study a sequence of martingales $M^{(n)}$, indexed by n. Let $M_\epsilon^{(n)}$ be a martingale containing all jumps of $M^{(n)}$ larger than ϵ in absolute value, and let the function $m(u)$ be a continuous increasing deterministic function.

Theorem 9.3 *Assume that* $[M^{(n)}]_u \xrightarrow{P} m(u)$ *or* $\langle M^{(n)} \rangle_u \xrightarrow{P} m(u)$ *and that for each* $\epsilon >$ 0, $M_\epsilon^{(n)}(u) \xrightarrow{P} 0$ *for all* u. *Then* $M^{(n)} \Rightarrow M^{(\infty)}$, *where* $M^{(\infty)}$ *is a continuous Gaussian martingale with* $\langle M^{(\infty)} \rangle_u = [M^{(\infty)}]_u = m(u)$. *In particular* $M^{(\infty)}(t) - M^{(\infty)}(s)$ *is Gaussian with mean 0 and variance* $m(t) - m(s)$ *for* $t \geq s$.

We omit the proof of the theorem. In the Markovian case it can be proven using methods similar to those presented in Chapter 5.

9.2 ML-estimation for the standard SIR epidemic

Assume now that we observe $E_{n,m}(\lambda, I)$ up to some time u, that is we observe all infection times τ_i and removal times ρ_i that have occurred up until u. Define $N_1(t) = n - X(t)$, a counting process for the number of infections that have occurred in $(0, t]$, and $N_2(t) = n + m - (X(t) + Y(t))$ a counting process for the number of removals in $(0, t]$ (remember that $X(0) = n$ and $Y(0) = m = \mu n$). The first counting process has intensity $(\lambda/n)X(t-)Y(t-)$. The counting process N_2 has a more complicated intensity. If F denotes the distribution of the infectious period I and f its density function then the intensity function at t is $\sum_i f(t-\tau_i)/(1-F(t-\tau_i))$, where the sum extends over individuals which are infectious at $t-$. Applying results of the previous section and manipulating the integrals for the counting process N_2 it follows that the log-likelihood is given by

$$\begin{aligned} \ell_u(\lambda, F) &= \int_0^u (\log[(\lambda/n)X(t-)Y(t-)]dN_1(t) - (\lambda/n)X(t-)Y(t-)dt) \\ &\quad + \sum_{i;\tau_i \leq u < \rho_i} \log(1 - F(u - \tau_i)) + \sum_{i;\rho_i \leq u} \log f(\rho_i - \tau_i). \end{aligned} \tag{9.4}$$

To estimate λ we differentiate the log-likelihood with respect to λ

$$\frac{\partial}{\partial \lambda}\ell_u(\lambda, F) = \int_0^u \frac{1}{\lambda}\left(dN_1(t) - \frac{\lambda}{n}X(t-)Y(t-)dt\right) = \frac{N_1(u)}{\lambda} - \int_0^u \bar{X}(t-)Y(t-)dt,$$

where, as before, $\bar{X}(t) = X(t)/n$. (Whenever integration is with respect to Lebesgue's measure (dt), as on the far right above, one may replace the argument '$t-$' by 't', this is done in what follows.) Solving the likelihood equation $\frac{\partial}{\partial \lambda}\ell_u(\lambda, F) = 0$ thus gives the ML-estimate

$$\hat{\lambda} = \frac{N_1(u)}{\int_0^u \bar{X}(t)Y(t)dt}. \tag{9.5}$$

Estimating properties of the infectious period can be done parametrically or non-parametrically. In particular, if the epidemic is observed to the end, $u = T = \inf\{t; Y(t) = 0\}$, then the first sum in (9.4) is empty and inference is based on the observed lengths of the infectious periods I_i among individuals who were infected. For example, $\iota = E[I]$ is simply estimated by the observed mean $\bar{I}$.

For the rest of this section we treat the Markovian version of the standard SIR model, i.e. assuming that the length of the infectious period is exponentially distributed with mean length $1/\gamma$. The reason for doing this is that convergence results can be derived from the theory presented in Chapter 5, but most results are true for the general case. For the Markovian case the intensity for $N_2(t)$ is simply $\gamma Y(t)$ (each infectious individual is removed at constant rate γ). The derivative of the likelihood with respect to γ then becomes

$$\frac{\partial}{\partial\gamma}\ell_u(\lambda,\gamma) = \int_0^u \frac{1}{\gamma}\left(dN_2(t) - \gamma Y(t)dt\right) = \frac{N_2(u)}{\gamma} - \int_0^u Y(t)dt.$$

Consequently, the ML estimator is

$$\hat{\gamma} = \frac{N_2(u)}{\int_0^u Y(t)dt}. \tag{9.6}$$

A more natural parameter to estimate is $1/\gamma$, the expected length of the infectious period, which is of course estimated by the inverse of the estimator above. In particular, if the epidemic is observed to the the end $u = T$ the estimator is $\int_0^T Y(t)dt/N_2(T)$, and this is simply the aggregated length of all infectious periods divided by the number who were removed. The estimator is hence simply the arithmetic mean of the observed infectious periods.

We will now prove that the ML-estimators are asymptotically normal. First we apply the martingale central limit theorem to the score processes.

Lemma 9.4 *Consider the Markovian version of the standard SIR epidemic with initial values $X^{(n)}(0) = n$ and $Y^{(n)}(0) = \mu n$. Define the normed score processes $S_1^{(n)}(u) = n^{-1/2}\frac{\partial}{\partial\lambda}\ell_u(\lambda,\gamma)$ and $S_2^{(n)}(u) = n^{-1/2}\frac{\partial}{\partial\gamma}\ell_u(\lambda,\gamma)$, evcluated at the true parameter values (λ_0,γ_0). Then*

$$S_1^{(n)} \Rightarrow S_1 \qquad \text{and} \qquad S_2^{(n)} \Rightarrow S_2,$$

where S_1 and S_2 are Gaussian martingales. The covariance function of S_1 and S_2, denoted v_1 and v_2 respectively, are defined through the deterministic limiting functions $x(t)$ and $y(t)$ of Section 5.5, and are given by

$$\begin{aligned} v_1(u) &= \lambda_0^{-2}\int_0^u \lambda_0 x(t)y(t)dt = \lambda_0^{-2}\left(1 - x(u)\right) \\ v_2(u) &= \gamma_0^{-2}\int_0^u \gamma_0 y(t)dt = \gamma_0^{-2}\left(1 + \mu - x(u) - y(u)\right), \end{aligned}$$

respectively.

Proof. The result follows immediately from the martingale central limit theorem (Theorem 9.3). The first assumption of the theorem was shown in Section 5.5, and since the size of all jumps are $n^{-1/2}$ for the normed process, there will be no jumps larger than ϵ for n large enough. •

We are now able to prove the main result of this chapter, a result originally given by Rida (1991).

Theorem 9.5 *The ML-estimators $\hat{\lambda}$ and $\hat{\gamma}$ are asymptotically Gaussian with asymptotic means λ_0 and γ_0 (the true parameter values) respectively. The asymptotic variance of $\hat{\lambda}$ is $1/nv_1(u)$ and for $\hat{\gamma}$ the variance is $1/nv_2(u)$. Consistent estimates of the standard errors of $\hat{\lambda}$ and the more natural parameter $\widehat{\gamma^{-1}} = 1/\hat{\gamma}$ (the average length of the infectious period) are*

$$\begin{aligned} \text{s.e.}\left(\hat{\lambda}\right) &= \hat{\lambda}/\sqrt{N_1(u)} \qquad \textit{and} \\ \text{s.e.}\left(\widehat{\gamma^{-1}}\right) &= \widehat{\gamma^{-1}}/\sqrt{N_2(u)}. \end{aligned}$$

For the case where the epidemic is observed to its end ($u = T$) the deterministic integrals appearing in the variance functions v_1 and v_2 may be replaced by $\tau - \mu$ and τ respectively (τ was defined in Chapter 4). Similarly, the square root expressions for the standard errors then becomes Z and $Z + \mu n$ respectively.

Proof. We prove the statement for $\hat{\lambda}$, the proof for $\hat{\gamma}$ being similar. The estimator $\hat{\lambda}$ is the solution to the likelihood equation $\frac{\partial}{\partial\lambda}\ell_u(\lambda,\gamma) = 0$. Multiplying the likelihood equation by $\lambda_0/\sqrt{n}$ gives

$$0 = \frac{1}{\sqrt{n}}\left(N_1(u) - \int_0^u \hat{\lambda}\bar{X}(t)Y(t)dt\right) = \lambda_0 S_1^{(n)}(u) + \frac{1}{\sqrt{n}}(\lambda_0 - \hat{\lambda})\int_0^u \bar{X}(t)Y(t)dt.$$

Rearranging the formula yields

$$\sqrt{n}\left(\hat{\lambda} - \lambda_0\right) = \frac{S_1^{(n)}(u)}{\lambda_0^{-1}\int_0^u \bar{X}(t)\bar{Y}(t)dt}. \tag{9.7}$$

According to Lemma 9.4 $S_1^{(n)}(u)$ converges to a Gaussian random variable with mean 0 and variance $v_1(u)$. Further, by Theorem 5.2 $\lambda_0^{-1}\int_0^u \bar{X}(t)\bar{Y}(t)dt$ converges in probability to $\int_0^u x(t)y(t)dt = v_1(u)$. Hence, by Slutsky's theorem it follows that $\hat{\lambda}$ is asymptotically normal with prescribed mean and variance. That $\int_0^\infty \lambda_0 x(t)y(t)dt = \tau - \mu$ is easily shown from the deterministic equations in Section 5.5. Finally, $\bar{N}_1(u)$ also converges in probability to $\int_0^u \lambda_0 x(t)y(t)dt$ using Theorem 5.2, from which it follows that the standard error is consistent. •

Of course, the basic reproduction number $\theta_0 = \lambda_0/\gamma_0$ is estimated by $\hat{\theta} = \hat{\lambda}/\hat{\gamma}$, where $\hat{\lambda}$ and $\hat{\gamma}$ are defined by (9.5) and (9.6) respectively. This estimator is also asymptotically Gaussian as the following corollary shows.

Corollary 9.6 *The estimator* $\hat{\theta} = \hat{\lambda}/\hat{\gamma}$ *is asymptotically Gaussian with mean* θ_0 *and variance* $\left(v_1^{-1}(u) + \theta_0^2 v_2^{-1}(u)\right)/(n\gamma_0^2)$. *If the epidemic is observed to its end (i.e.* $u = T$*) then a consistent standard error is given by* $\text{s.e.}(\hat{\theta}) = \hat{\theta}\sqrt{\left(\bar{Z}^{-1} + (\bar{Z}+\mu)^{-1}\right)/n}$.

Proof. The proof consists of two steps. First we argue that $\hat{\lambda}$ and $\hat{\gamma}$ are asymptotically independent. The second part, left for Exercise 9.2, consists of applying the δ-method, i.e. expanding $\hat{\lambda}$ and $\hat{\gamma}$ around their true values λ_0 and γ_0, by Taylor's theorem, and using their independence. To show that $\hat{\lambda}$ and $\hat{\gamma}$ are asymptotically independent we note that, by definition $\sqrt{n}\left(\hat{\gamma}^{-1} - \gamma_0^{-1}\right) = S_2^{(n)}(u)/\bar{N}_2(u)$ and a similar expression for $\sqrt{n}\left(\hat{\lambda} - \lambda_0\right)$ is given in Equation (9.7). The denominators in the two expressions converge in probability to deterministic limits, and $S_1^{(n)}$ and $S_2^{(n)}$ are uncorrelated due to Lemma 9.2 which proves asymptotic independence. •

Statistical analysis for various extensions of the standard SIR model, assuming complete observation, has not received much attention in the literature. One reason for this is that the epidemic process is rarely observed in such detail. Another reason is that for many models (e.g. most network models) stochastic properties of the epidemic process are unknown, only properties of the final state having been derived. Two exceptions are Rhodes *et al.* (1996) and Britton (1998a). The former considers a more detailed model for a homogeneous community and assumes even more detailed data; information about actual contacts is known. For such data Rhodes *et al.* (1996) derive estimation procedures for various parameters, including the probability that a contact leads to infection. Britton (1998a) derives estimation procedures based on complete data for the Markovian version of the multitype epidemic model (see Chapter 6). It is shown that the infectivity of a given type can only be estimated consistently if the corresponding susceptibility differs from all other susceptibilities.

Exercises

9.1. Prove Lemma 9.2. (Hint: Use the same technique as in the proof of Lemma 9.1, i.e. to divide the interval into small disjoint intervals of length h and show that the conditional expectation of each term is 0, the diagonal terms as well! To be precise the terms are of order $o(h^2)$.)

9.2. Prove the remaining part of Corollary 9.6. (Hint: Apply the δ-method together with the results of Theorem 9.5 and independence to derive the asymptotic variance of the estimator $\hat{\theta}$.)

9.3. Table 9.1 on the next two pages describes an outbreak of smallpox in a Nigerian village (taken from Table 6.1 p 112-113, Becker, 1989). For each day the number of susceptibles and infectives are given as well as the number of infections that occurred during that day. (Note that the number of infectives does not increase as soon as an infection occurs. The reason for this is that individuals are latent for some time before turning susceptible. This does not affect estimates.) Assume this to be an outbreak from the Markovian version of $E_{n,m}(\lambda, I)$.

a) Estimate the infection parameter λ, the mean length of the infectious period γ^{-1} and the basic reproduction number $\theta = \lambda/\gamma$.

b) Give standard errors for the estimates.

9.4. Suppose that instead of having $X(0) = n$ we have $X(0) = sn$, meaning that only a proportion s of those not initially infectious are susceptible and the remaining are immune (if the number of removed is denoted $Z(t)$ we hence have $Z(0) = (1-s)n$ under the present assumption). What is the effect on the ML-estimator $\hat{\lambda}$ and its variance? Answer the question by considering two communities having the same *numbers* of infectives and susceptibles initially and all through the epidemic, only one community having no initially immune and the other community having, say, half as many initially immune as initially susceptible. (Hint: Note that the two communities have different $n = X(0) + Z(0)$).

Table 9.1. The spread of smallpox in a Nigerian village (continued)

Time t	Number infectious $I(t)$	Number suscept. $S(t)$	Number infected $C(t)$	Time t	Number infectious $I(t)$	Number suscept. $S(t)$	Number infected $C(t)$
0	1	119	1	22	1	111	1
1	1	118	0	23	2	110	0
2	1	118	0	24	2	110	0
3	1	118	0	25	2	110	1
4	1	118	0	26	5	109	0
5	1	118	0	27	6	109	2
6	1	118	0	28	5	107	0
7	1	118	1	29	5	107	2
8	1	117	0	30	4	105	0
9	1	117	1	31	5	105	0
10	1	116	0	32	5	105	0
11	1	116	0	33	2	105	0
12	1	116	3	34	1	105	1
13	1	113	1	35	1	104	0
14	1	112	0	36	2	104	0
15	1	112	0	37	2	104	1
16	1	112	0	38	1	103	1
17	1	112	1	39	2	102	0
18	1	111	0	40	2	102	0
19	1	111	0	41	4	102	0
20	1	111	0	42	4	102	2
21	1	111	0	43	5	100	1

Time t	Number infectious $I(t)$	Number suscept. $S(t)$	Number infected $C(t)$	Time t	Number infectious $I(t)$	Number susceptib. $S(t)$	Number infected $C(t)$
44	5	99	1	64	5	90	0
45	5	98	1	65	4	90	0
46	4	97	0	66	3	90	0
47	4	97	2	67	5	90	0
48	3	95	1	68	3	90	0
49	3	94	0	69	2	90	0
50	1	94	0	70	2	90	0
51	2	94	0	71	2	90	0
52	3	94	0	72	3	90	0
53	3	94	2	73	3	90	0
54	3	92	0	74	1	90	0
55	2	92	0	75	1	90	0
56	4	92	0	76	1	90	0
57	5	92	0	77	2	90	0
58	5	92	1	78	2	90	0
59	5	91	0	79	1	90	0
60	5	91	0	80	1	90	0
61	7	91	0	81	1	90	0
62	8	91	0	82	1	90	0
63	6	91	1	83	1	90	0

10 Estimation in partially observed epidemics

In the previous chapter, statistical analysis was based on what we called complete observation of the epidemic process; both the times of infection and removal (recovery) for all infected individuals were observed. In real life such detailed data is rarely available. In the present chapter we study estimation procedures for less detailed partial data. The likelihood for partial data is usually cumbersome to work with, being a sum or integral over all complete data sets resulting in the observed partial data. Other estimation techniques can turn out to be much simpler. Below we present two general techniques which have been successful in several epidemic applications: martingale methods and the EM-algorithm.

The two techniques are applied to a specific estimation problem. First, we use martingale methods to derive an estimator for the basic reproduction number in the standard SIR epidemic, assuming that only the initial and final states are observed. Second, we consider a discrete time version of the models presented previously, introducing chain-binomial models, which are interesting in their own right. Assuming that the chains are observed we make use of the EM-algorithm to deduce an estimator of the transmission parameter. It is worth pointing out that pure likelihood methods *can* be applied in several cases, even when only partial data is available. If, for example, several small sub-populations (e.g. households) are observed, then ML-estimation is often possible from final size data. Estimation then consists of traditional ML-theory with the additional ingredient of potential numerical problems due to the complicated form of the likelihood (cf. the exact likelihood in Section 2.4). Addy *et al.* (1991) present estimation procedures for final size data of sub-populations, allowing for a heterogeneous community and also for transmission from outside the sub-population. The ideas extend the early work by Longini and Koopman (1982) who treat a homogeneous community and a special form of transmission dynamics.

10.1 Estimation based on martingale methods

The standard SIR epidemic $E_{n,m}(\lambda, I)$ was defined in Section 2.1. Suppose that we have collected data from such an epidemic and that data consist of knowing how many individuals have been infected during the course of the epidemic, besides knowing the initial state (i.e. the number of initially susceptible and infectious individuals respectively). In many cases the initial state may not be known. The initial number of infectives is usually small thus not causing much uncertainty; the substantial problem lies in knowing how many individuals are initially susceptible to the disease. Quite often some individuals are immune even before the disease is introduced, perhaps due to an earlier outbreak of the same or a similar disease. Then the number of susceptibles has to be estimated prior to the outbreak, using traditional statistical methods. Here we assume this number to be known thus neglecting such uncertainty.

Our data consists of $n = X(0)$, $\mu n = Y(0)$ (the initial state) and the final number infected $Z = n - X(T)$, and implicitly knowing that $Y(T) = 0$ since there are are no infectious individuals at the end of the epidemic. As observed in Section 2.4 the exact distribution of the final size of the epidemic has a numerically complicated form, thus not enabling much help in estimation when n is large. One way to estimate is of course to use the central limit theorem stating that Z is approximately normally distributed and equating the mean to the observed value Z. Here we take a different approach based on martingale methods, a method applicable in many other cases.

From Chapter 9 we know that

$$\int_0^u f(t)\left(dN_1(t) - \lambda_0 \bar{X}(t)Y(t)dt\right) - \int_0^u g(t)\left(dN_2(t) - \gamma_0 Y(t)dt\right)$$

is a martingale for any choice of predictable (left-continuous) processes $f = \{f(t); t \geq 0\}$ and $g = \{g(t); t \geq 0\}$. The ML-estimator $\hat{\lambda}$ was obtained by equating the martingale to 0 for the choice $f(t) = 1/\lambda$ and $g(t) = 0$, and $\hat{\gamma}$ from $f(t) = 0$ and $g(t) = 1/\gamma$. This method can no longer be used in the case of final size data: for example $\int_0^u \bar{X}(t)Y(t)dt$ appearing in $\hat{\lambda}$ is not observed. However, the same idea of equating a martingale to its mean, a special form of the method of moments, can be adopted by choosing f and g cleverly so that the resulting martingale only depends on observed quantities. We want to choose f and g such that the 'dt' terms cancel out. This happens if $f(t) = \gamma_0/(\lambda_0\bar{X}(t-))$ (note that $f(t)$ is left-continuous) and $g(t) = 1$. Let $M^{(n)}$ denote the resulting zero-mean martingale divided by $\sqrt{n}$ and let $\theta_0 = \lambda_0/\gamma_0$ be the basic reproduction number. That is,

$$\begin{aligned}
\sqrt{n}M^{(n)}(u) &= \int_0^u \frac{1}{\theta_0\bar{X}(t-)}\left(dN_1(t) - \lambda_0\bar{X}(t)Y(t)dt\right) - \int_0^u \left(dN_2(t) - \gamma_0 Y(t)dt\right)\\
&= \frac{1}{\theta_0}\int_0^u \frac{1}{\bar{X}(t-)}dN_1(t) - \int_0^u dN_2(t)\\
&= \frac{n}{\theta_0}\left(\frac{1}{n} + \frac{1}{n-1} + \cdots + \frac{1}{n-(N_1(u)-1)}\right) - N_2(u).
\end{aligned} \qquad (10.1)$$

The last equality is true since $X(t) = n - N_1(t)$. For $u = T$, the end of the epidemic, its value is determined by the final size data since $N_1(T) = Z$ and $N_2(T) = \mu n + Z$. Solving the equation $M^{(n)}(T) = 0$ leads to the estimator

$$\hat{\hat{\theta}} = \frac{\frac{1}{n} + \frac{1}{n-1} + \cdots + \frac{1}{n-(Z-1)}}{\bar{Z} + \mu}. \qquad (10.2)$$

To see that the estimator is reasonable, we look at its large population approximation using the approximation $1/n + 1/(n-1) + \cdots + 1/(n-(Z-1)) \approx -\log(1-\bar{Z})$ implying that

$$\hat{\hat{\theta}} \approx -\log(1-\bar{Z})/(\bar{Z}+\mu).$$

From the law of large numbers derived in Section 4.3 it is seen that the estimator agrees with the large population limit. The large population limit for $\bar{Z}+\mu$, denoted by τ, is defined in (4.1), where $\iota = E(I)$ corresponds to $1/\gamma_0$ (and hence $\lambda\iota$ to θ_0) for the Markovian case treated here.

A central limit theorem can be derived using methods similar to those in the case of complete data treated in Section 9.2. From the martingale central limit theorem (Theorem 9.3) we have the following corollary:

Corollary 10.1 *The martingale $M^{(n)}$ defined by (10.1) satisfies $M^{(n)} \Rightarrow M$. The limiting process M is a continuous Gaussian martingale with covariance function*

$$v(u) = \frac{1}{\theta_0^2}\left(\frac{1}{x(u)} - 1\right) + (1+\mu - x(u) - y(u)),$$

where $x(u)$ and $y(u)$ are deterministic functions defined in Section 5.5. The martingale observed at its end, $M^{(n)}(T) = M^{(n)}(\infty)$, converges to a Gaussian random variable with mean 0 and variance $v(\infty) = \theta_0^{-2}\left((1+\mu-\tau)^{-1} - 1\right) + \tau$.

Proof. The optional variation process $[M^{(n)}]$ has the following form

$$\begin{aligned}[M^{(n)}]_u &= \frac{1}{n\theta_0^2}\int_0^u \frac{1}{\bar{X}^2(t-)} dN_1(t) + \frac{1}{n}\int_0^u dN_2(t) \\ &= \frac{1}{n\theta_0^2}\left(1 + \frac{1}{(1-1/n)^2} + \cdots + \frac{1}{(\bar{X}(u)+1/n)^2}\right) + (1+\mu-\bar{X}(u)-\bar{Y}(u)).\end{aligned}$$

(The fact the N_1 and N_2 jump at distinct time-points makes the two martingales defined from N_1 and N_2 independent, cf. Lemma 9.2, so the variation process of their difference is the sum of the two variation processes.) From Chapter 5 we know that $\bar{X}(u)$ and $\bar{Y}(u)$ respectively converge to $x(u)$ and $y(u)$ of Section 5.5 almost surely, uniformly on bounded intervals. Because an integral is defined as the limit of a sum with smaller and smaller time increments it then follows that $[M^{(n)}]_u$ converges to $v(u)$. Because the jumps of $M^{(n)}$ are of size $1/\sqrt{n}$ we can then apply Theorem 9.3 to conclude weak convergence of the martingale. A formal proof of the final statement is technical and not given here (see Rida, 1991). The variance is as expected since $x(\infty) = 1+\mu-\tau$ and $y(\infty) = 0$, the asymptotic proportions of susceptibles and infectives respectively at the end of the epidemic. •

The corollary above immediately induces a central limit theorem for the estimator $\hat{\hat{\theta}}$ which we state in the following corollary (see also Rida, 1991).

Corollary 10.2 *The estimator $\hat{\hat{\theta}}$ defined in (10.2) is asymptotically normally distributed with mean θ_0 and asymptotic variance*

$$\frac{1}{n\tau^2}\left(\frac{\tau-\mu}{1-(\tau-\mu)} + \theta_0^2\tau\right)$$

where τ is defined in (4.1) with θ_0 replacing $\lambda\iota$. A consistent standard error for the estimator is given by

$$\text{s.e.}(\hat{\hat{\theta}}) = \frac{1}{\sqrt{n}(\bar{Z}+\mu)}\left(\frac{\bar{Z}}{1-\bar{Z}} + \hat{\hat{\theta}}^2(\bar{Z}+\mu)\right)^{1/2}.$$

Proof. From the definition of $\hat{\hat{\theta}}$ we have

$$0 = \sqrt{n}M^{(n)}(T) + \left(\frac{1}{\hat{\hat{\theta}}} - \frac{1}{\theta_0}\right)\int_0^T \frac{1}{\bar{X}(t-)}dN_1(t).$$

Rearranging the formula gives $\theta_0^{-1} - \hat{\hat{\theta}}^{-1} = \sqrt{n}M^{(n)}(T)/\int_0^T \bar{X}(t)^{-1}dN_1(t)$. As noted earlier, the integral equals $n\left(1/n + \cdots + 1/(n-Z+1)\right)$. In Section 4.2 it was shown that Z/n converges in probability to $\tau - \mu$. Hence it follows that

$$\frac{1}{n} + \cdots + \frac{1}{n-Z+1} \to -\log(1+\mu-\tau)$$

in probability, and the right hand side is equal to $\theta_0\tau$ due to the definition of τ. Together with Corollary 10.1, stating that $M^{(n)}(T)$ is asymptotically normal we can apply Slutsky's theorem to conclude that $\sqrt{n}(\theta_0^{-1} - \hat{\hat{\theta}}^{-1})$ converges to a Gaussian random variable with mean 0 and variance $(\theta_0\tau)^{-2}\left(\theta_0^{-2}\left((1+\mu-\tau)^{-1}-1\right)+\tau\right)$. Finally, apply the δ-method, i.e. derive the Taylor expansion of the estimator around the true parameter, to conclude that asymptotically $\text{Var}(\hat{\hat{\theta}}) = \theta_0^4\text{Var}(\hat{\hat{\theta}}^{-1})$. •

Using martingale methods we have shown how to derive an estimator for θ based on observing only the final size. If the complete data were available a better estimator is of course $\hat{\theta} = \hat{\lambda}/\hat{\gamma}$ of Chapter 9, which uses more information. When only the final size is observed we cannot estimate the two parameters separately. This is quite natural: one random quantity (the final size) enables estimation of one parameter, and since we have no knowledge of the time evolution of the process, we should not expect any information about the length of the infectious period.

Sometimes information about the time of diagnosis of infected individuals is also available. The time of diagnosis is approximately equal to the 'removal time' because social activity is often reduced when symptoms become obvious, and so is the infectiousness. This motivates the study by Becker and Hasofer (1997), which derives estimation procedures for data on removal times, assuming the Markovian version of the standard SIR epidemic. Besides the martingale considered above, they derive another estimating equation from the martingale $\tilde{M}(t) = X(t)(1+\theta/n)^{n+\mu n - X(t) - Y(t)}$. This enables them to estimate λ and γ separately as in the case of complete data.

Britton (1998a) has constructed estimators, using martingale methods similar to those of the present section, for final size data of the multitype SIR model of

Chapter 6, assuming proportionate mixing. Susceptibility parameters are shown to be asymptotically Gaussian whereas infectivities and the basic reproduction number cannot be estimated consistently. An explanation is that the dimension of the data is lower than the number of parameters, and by observing those who were infected, not much can be said about those who caused the disease to spread further, i.e. about the infectivities.

10.2 Estimation based on the EM-algorithm

The EM-algorithm was first named by Dempster, Laird and Rubin (1977), but the method dates back even earlier. It is a method aiming at simplifying likelihood inference by introducing more detailed hypothetical data. First, we explain the general method very briefly, and then give an application to epidemic inference.

Let x denote the observed data and suppose we wish to estimate some parameter(s) θ, but that the log-likelihood $\ell(\theta; x)$ is cumbersome to work with. Suppose further that estimation would be much simpler, or even trivial, if some hypothetical data y, containing x, were available. The EM-algorithm then suggests that one 'pretend' this more detailed data is available and estimate the parameter(s). Then one computes the expected value of the hypothetical data given the observed data. This algorithm is repeated until the change in value of the parameter estimate is negligible. Using mathematical notation one should start with an initial parameter choice $\theta_{(0)}$. Then perform the E(xpectation)-step and M(aximization)-step repeatedly, where the E- and M-steps respectively consist of computing

$$\begin{aligned} \text{E-step} &: \; f(\theta; x, \theta_{(j-1)}) = E(\ell(\theta; Y)|x; \theta_{(j-1)}) \\ \text{M-step} &: \; \theta_{(j)} = \text{argmax}_\theta f(\theta; x, \theta_{(j-1)}). \end{aligned}$$

This algorithm is iterated until the difference between $\theta_{(j)}$ and $\theta_{(j+1)}$ is negligible. The resulting value is the parameter estimate. The hard part of the EM-algorithm lies in inventing suitable imaginary data. How this is done varies from application to application.

We now apply this method to an estimation problem in epidemics, where we consider a discrete time epidemic model within the class of chain-binomial models. For each integer k, let X_k and Y_k respectively denote the number of susceptible and infectious individuals at time, or generation, k. The name chain-binomial comes from the way susceptible individuals are reduced (i.e. become infected): given $X_k = x_k$ and $Y_k = y_k$ the number of susceptible individuals at $k+1$, X_{k+1}, is binomially distributed with parameters x_k and q^{y_k}. This means that a susceptible individual in generation k remains susceptible at $k+1$ if she escapes infection from each of the y_k infectious individuals at k, and these non-infective events are independent and occur with probability q. Here we concentrate on estimation of q based on the data $(x_1, y_1), \ldots, (x_r, y_r)$; we do not have to consider how long individuals are in the latent state and infectious before becoming removed. The simplest and most studied model is known as the discrete time Reed-Frost model where it is assumed that the infected individuals become infectious immediately and are removed in the next generation implying that $y_{k+1} = x_k - x_{k+1}$. All we assume here is that infections occur according to the chain-binomial model. We therefore introduce the notation $i_{k+1} = x_k - x_{k+1}$ to denote the number of individuals that become infected in generation $k+1$, contained in the data.

The likelihood with respect to q of the data is

$$\prod_{k=1}^{r-1} \binom{x_k}{x_{k+1}} (q^{y_k})^{x_{k+1}} (1 - q^{y_k})^{i_{k+1}},$$

and the log-likelihood is given by

$$\ell(q; \{x_k, y_k\}) = c + \sum_{k=1}^{r-1} (x_{k+1} \log(q^{y_k}) + i_{k+1} \log(1 - q^{y_k})).$$

To maximize this expression is numerically complicated if the number of infectious individuals is high in some generations. The reason is that the derivative of the second term above then becomes messy. Suppose that rather than observing (x_{k+1}, i_{k+1}) we observed $x_{k+1,0}, x_{k+1,1}, \ldots, x_{k+1,y_k}$, where $x_{k+1,j}$ is the number of individuals susceptible in generation k who had j (out of y_k) infectious contacts. Note that $\sum_{j\geq 1} x_{k+1,j} = i_{k+1}$ and $x_{k+1,0} = x_{k+1}$. This data extension separates the probability $(1 - q^{y_k})$ into the terms $\binom{y_k}{j}(1-q)^j q^{y_k - j}$. Estimation of this extended model is close to trivial. The log-likelihood is given by

$$\ell(q; \{x_{k,0}, x_{k,1}, \ldots, x_{k,y_{k-1}}, y_k\}) = c + \sum_{k=1}^{r-1} \sum_{j=0}^{y_k} x_{k+1,j} \, (j \log(1-q) + (y_k - j) \log q).$$

Differentiating this and equating the likelihood equation to 0 reveals that the ML-estimator for the extended data is

$$\hat{q} = \frac{\sum_{k=1}^{r-1} \sum_{j=0}^{y_k} (y_k - j) x_{k+1,j}}{\sum_{k=1}^{r-1} \sum_{j=0}^{y_k} y_k x_{k+1,j}} = \frac{\sum_{k=1}^{r-1} y_k x_k - \sum_{k=1}^{r-1} \sum_{j=0}^{y_k} j x_{k+1,j}}{\sum_{k=1}^{r-1} y_k x_k}.$$

Note that the estimator is simply the number of contacts *not* resulting in infection divided by the total number of contacts. Unfortunately the data $x_{k+1,1}, \ldots, x_{k+1,y_k}$ is not available. We therefore replace the unobserved quantities above by their expected values given the available data. For $j \geq 1$ we have

$$E[X_{k+1,j} | \{x_k, y_k\}; q] = i_{k+1} \frac{\binom{y_k}{j}(1-q)^j q^{y_k - j}}{1 - q^{y_k}}.$$

This follows because each of the y_k individuals who were infected has a binomially distributed number of infectious contacts, a number conditioned on being positive.

The expectation of the negative term in the numerator of $\hat{q}$ is therefore $\sum_k i_{k+1}(1-q)y_k/(1-q^{y_k})$.

The EM-algorithm starts with an initial guess $q_{(0)}$ and then updates the estimate iteratively according to the iteration function

$$q_{(j)} = 1 - \frac{\sum_{k=1}^{r-1} i_{k+1} \frac{(1-q_{(j-1)})y_k}{1-q_{(j-1)}^{y_k}}}{\sum_{k=1}^{r-1} y_k x_k}.$$

Iterating this function is very easy, since only the numerator has to be re-evaluated each iteration. In practice less than 10 iterations should suffice for the estimator to converge.

The EM-algorithm has been used successfully in many areas of statistics. In the analysis of infectious disease data it seems suitable for several problems but often methods remain to be developed. In Becker (1997) the EM-algorithm is applied to several problems, with a particular interest in HIV/AIDS data.

Exercises

10.1. Consider the data in Exercise 9.3 and adopt the same model assumptions. Estimate θ and give the standard error assuming only the final state is observed.

10.2. During October/November 1967 an outbreak of respiratory disease occurred on the isolated island of Tristan da Cunha (see Section 8.2.3 of Becker, 1989, for more details on on the data). Among the 255 individuals of the island 40 infections occurred. Assume that one individual was infected from outside and that all other individuals were susceptible to the disease (reasonable assumption). Estimate θ and derive the standard error for the estimate under the simplifying assumption of a homogeneous uniformly mixing population).

10.3. The standard deviation of $\hat{\theta}$ based on complete observation of the epidemic process should be smaller than the standard deviation of $\hat{\hat{\theta}}$, but how much? Derive an expression for the ratio of the standard errors for the final size and complete data estimators. Compute the ratio numerically for $\theta_0 = 1.5$ and $\theta_0 = 2.5$. (Hint: Use the expressions for the standard errors in Corollaries 9.6 and 10.2 and their large population limits.)

10.4. Prove that $\tilde{M}(t) = X(t)(1+\theta/n)^{n+\mu n - X(t) - Y(t)}$ is a martingale (this martingale is used by Becker and Hasofer, 1997, to construct an estimating equation). (Hint: Look at a small time increment $\tilde{M}(t+h) - M(t)$ and show that its expectation, conditioned on $X(t)$ and $Y(t)$, equals 0.)

10.5. Table 10.1 below describes an outbreak of common cold in 664 households of size 5 (taken from Table 2.7, p 31, Becker, 1989). Each household has one introductory case, after this external infections can be neglected. Infections are observed in terms of generations and infected individuals become infectious immediately and remain so over one generation only (this implies that $y_k = i_k$ using the notation of Section 10.2). A chain $1 \to 2 \to 1$ hence implies that ($y_1 = 1$, $x_1 = 4$), $y_2 = 2$, $x_2 = 2$, $y_3 = 1$, $x_3 = 1$ and $y_4 = 0$, $x_4 = 1$ for this household. Use the EM-algorithm to estimate q, the probability to escape infection from one infectious individual over one generation. (When estimating q you should use all households by treating each chain separately. That is, in the iterative estimator $q_{(k)}$ you should sum also over all households.) You may of course use exact ML estimates if you prefer.

Table 10.1. Outbreak chains for common cold in households of size 5

Chain	Obs. frequency
1	423
$1 \to 1$	131
$1 \to 1 \to 1$	36
$1 \to 2$	24
$1 \to 1 \to 1 \to 1$	14
$1 \to 1 \to 2$	8
$1 \to 2 \to 1$	11
$1 \to 3$	3
$1 \to 1 \to 1 \to 1 \to 1$	4
$1 \to 1 \to 1 \to 2$	2
$1 \to 1 \to 2 \to 1$	2
$1 \to 1 \to 3$	2
$1 \to 2 \to 1 \to 1$	3
$1 \to 2 \to 2$	1
$1 \to 3 \to 1$	0
$1 \to 4$	0

11 Markov Chain Monte Carlo

Markov Chain Monte Carlo (MCMC) is a computer-intensive statistical tool that has received considerable attention over the past few years. Using MCMC theory, it is often quite simple to write efficient algorithms for sampling from extremely complicated target distributions; thus, it is not difficult to understand why these techniques have found important applications in a vast number of different areas. Although the literature on MCMC methods is growing rapidly, the excellent book by Gilks, Richardson and Spiegelhalter (1996) provides a good starting point for the interested reader.

In the first two sections of this chapter we present the main ideas of MCMC, and apply the techniques to two important situations: Calculating expectations with respect to complicated probability measures, and optimizing complicated functions. The optimization method described can sometimes be a good alternative to the EM-algorithm for calculating ML-estimators, but this point will not be developed further here. In Section 11.3 some practical issues are discussed, regarding e.g. convergence diagnostics. Finally, in Section 11.4 we describe a Bayesian approach for drawing inferences about basic parameters in stochastic epidemic models of the SIR type. (Most current applications of MCMC are oriented towards Bayesian inference, as are also those in the epidemic area. The example described here is taken from O'Neill and Roberts, 1999, but see also O'Neill *et al.*, 199?.)

11.1 Description of the techniques

The idea which lies behind Markov Chain Monte Carlo, first introduced by Metropolis *et al.* (1953), is in fact very simple. Suppose that we wish to sample from some target distribution $\pi(x)$, $x \in E \subseteq \mathbf{R}^p$, which is known only up to some multiplicative constant. In situations where π is sufficiently complex so that simple Monte Carlo methods cannot be used, an indirect sampling method would be to construct an aperiodic and irreducible Markov chain with state space E whose stationary distribution is given by π. This means that after having run the chain to stationarity, we can extract a (dependent) sample of any desired size from the target distribution. Some important questions immediately present themselves:

- Is it always possible to construct a Markov chain with the desired properties?
- How do we find a suitable starting point?
- How do we determine the *burn-in* period, i.e. the number of iterations needed until the chain is sufficiently close to stationarity?
- What are the implications of the fact that there are dependencies in the sample?

We answer the first question right away, leaving the other issues until Section 11.3.

Constructing a Markov chain with state space E and stationary distribution π is surprisingly easy. We describe here the *Metropolis-Hastings algorithm* (see Hastings, 1970), an algorithm that is easy to understand and implement.

The Markov chain X_ν, $\nu = 0, 1, 2, \ldots$, is started at some suitable point in E. Given $X_\nu = x$, the next state $X_{\nu+1}$ is chosen by first sampling a *candidate* point Y from some *proposal* distribution $q(\cdot \mid x)$ and then accepting this candidate with probability $\alpha(x, Y)$, where

$$\alpha(x, y) = \min\left(1, \frac{\pi(y)q(x \mid y)}{\pi(x)q(y \mid x)}\right). \tag{11.1}$$

If Y is accepted then of course $X_{\nu+1} = Y$, otherwise $X_{\nu+1} = X_\nu$. As soon as a proposal distribution, suitable for the problem at hand, has been specified implementation of the Metropolis-Hastings algorithm is easy. Note that possibly nasty normalizing factors in the target distribution disappear, since only the ratio $\pi(y)/\pi(x)$ is needed in the calculation of the acceptance probability $\alpha(x, y)$.

We now argue that the distribution of X_ν converges to the target distribution π as $\nu \to \infty$. The transition probability is given by

$$P(y \mid x) = q(y \mid x)\alpha(x, y) \qquad \text{for all } y \neq x \text{ (acceptance)},$$

and

$$P(x \mid x) = 1 - \int q(y \mid x)\alpha(x, y)\, dy \qquad \text{(rejection)}.$$

By checking separately the cases where the quotient in (11.1) is below one and above one, respectively, it follows immediately that

$$\pi(x)q(y \mid x)\alpha(x, y) = \pi(y)q(x \mid y)\alpha(y, x),$$

implying *detailed balance* for the chain:

$$\pi(x)P(y \mid x) = \pi(y)P(x \mid y)$$

for all $x, y \in E$. Integrate both sides of the detailed balance equation with respect to x to obtain

$$\int \pi(x)P(y \mid x)\, dx = \pi(y)$$

for all $y \in E$. Thus π is stationary for the process X. Under weak regularity conditions on the proposal distribution it can be shown that X actually converges in distribution, regardless of the choice of initial value.

The performance of the algorithm depends heavily on the form of the proposal distribution q. For computational efficiency, q should be chosen so that it can be easily sampled and evaluated. On the other hand, q and π must be related in such a way that the acceptance probability α becomes reasonably large; otherwise the chain might be *mixing* slowly (i.e. moving slowly around the support of π).

Let us now briefly present three widely used updating schemes. The *Metropolis algorithm* assumes that $q(y \mid x) = q(x \mid y)$ for all $x, y \in E$. This is the case if e.g. the proposal only depends on the distance between the points x and y, $q(y \mid x) = q(|y-x|)$. Then the acceptance probability reduces to

$$\alpha(x, y) = \min\left(1, \frac{\pi(y)}{\pi(x)}\right).$$

Another simple updating scheme, called the *independence sampler*, is obtained by putting $q(y \mid x) = q(y)$, so that new candidate points are chosen without considering the present value of the chain. In this case,

$$\alpha(x, y) = \min\left(1, \frac{w(y)}{w(x)}\right),$$

where $w(x) = \pi(x)/q(x)$. For the independence sampler to work well, q should be a fairly good approximation to π.

Finally we describe the *Gibbs sampler*. Suppose that E is a subset of the possibly high-dimensional space $\mathbf{R}^p$. We run through the indices i, $1 \leq i \leq p$, sequentially, and for a given index i we choose $q(y \mid x)$ as follows:

$$q(y \mid x) = \pi(y_i \mid x_1 \cdots x_{i-1} x_{i+1} \cdots x_p)$$

if $y_j = x_j$ for all $j \neq i$, and $q(y \mid x) = 0$ otherwise. Thus the candidate point y is obtained by changing the ith coordinate of x according to the full conditional distribution. A quick calculation shows that $\alpha(x, y) = 1$ for all $x, y \in E$, meaning that new candidates are always accepted! The Gibbs sampler is particularly well suited to deal with spatial models, where the full conditional distribution of a single site often depends only on the nearest neighbouring sites and can consequently be written down easily.

11.2 Important examples

Calculating expectations

The problem of calculating expectations of complicated high-dimensional distributions arises in many situations. Let X be a random variable with distribution $\pi(x)$, $x \in E \subseteq \mathbf{R}^p$, and consider the expression

$$E[f(X)] = \int f(x)\pi(x)\, dx,$$

for some function f of interest. If it is possible to use classical Monte Carlo simulation to draw an independent sample X_ν, $1 \leq \nu \leq n$, with the correct distribution, then the time average

$$\frac{1}{n}\sum_{\nu=1}^{n} f(X_\nu) \tag{11.2}$$

is guaranteed to provide an accurate approximation of $E[f(X)]$ if only the sample size n is large enough. On the other hand, in cases where straightforward Monte Carlo methods fail, we may instead use MCMC to obtain a dependent sample X_ν, $1 \leq \nu \leq n$, and again form the time average (11.2). Under certain regularity conditions on the Markov chain (see e.g. Roberts and Smith, 1994), we may apply the *ergodic theorem* to show that the time average is consistent, i.e.

$$\frac{1}{n}\sum_{\nu=1}^{n} f(X_\nu) \to E[f(X)]$$

almost surely as $n \to \infty$. (A detailed presentation of ergodic theory lies beyond the scope of this text.) In practice, the values X_ν from the burn-in period are usually discarded when calculating time averages.

Stochastic annealing

We now turn to another topic, namely optimization of non-standard functions using MCMC techniques. We are faced with the problem of minimizing a real-valued function $f(x)$, $x \in E \subseteq \mathbf{R}^p$, where for simplicity it is assumed that E consists of all the integer vectors inside some large box. Thus, every point x in E (excluding the boundary) has $2p$ nearest neighbours in E. Also, the optimal point, $\hat{x}$ say, is *unique* by assumption. Implicitly we assume that there is no good deterministic algorithm available to lead us to the vicinity of the optimal point $\hat{x}$, as is often the case in real-life problems. We will demonstrate how a series of well chosen Metropolis algorithms can be used to solve the problem. The technique is known as *stochastic* (or *simulated*) *annealing*.

Given $\beta > 0$ we define the target distribution

$$\pi^\beta(x) = \frac{e^{-\beta f(x)}}{\sum_{y \in E} e^{-\beta f(y)}}, \qquad x \in E.$$

The following Markov chain X_ν^β, $\nu \geq 1$, will have π^β as its stationary distribution. Start anywhere in E. Given $X_\nu^\beta = x$, propose one of the nearest neighbours at random, and call this point Y. Then accept the new point with probability $\alpha^\beta(x, Y)$, where

$$\alpha^\beta(x, y) = \min\left(1, \frac{\pi^\beta(y)}{\pi^\beta(x)}\right) = \min\left(1, e^{-\beta[f(y)-f(x)]}\right).$$

It is easily checked that this updating scheme corresponds to the Metropolis algorithm described in the last section, hence the theory tells us that π^β is indeed the stationary distribution for X^β.

The trick is now to run through a sequence of Metropolis algorithms according to the following scheme:

- Take $\beta > 0$ and pick a starting point in E;
- Run X^β close to stationarity;
- Increase β by a small amount, $\beta \to \beta'$;
- With the old endpoint as starting point, run a new Markov chain $X^{\beta'}$ close to stationarity;
- Increase β' by a small amount, $\beta' \to \beta''$;

and so on. As β becomes large, π^β becomes more and more peaked at the optimal point $\hat{x}$, since

$$\pi^\beta(x) = \frac{e^{-\beta f(x)}}{\sum_{y \in E} e^{-\beta f(y)}} = \frac{e^{-\beta[f(x)-f(\hat{x})]}}{\sum_{y \in E} e^{-\beta[f(y)-f(\hat{x})]}},$$

which tends to 1 as $\beta \to \infty$ if $x = \hat{x}$, and otherwise tends to 0. This indicates that a carefully tuned stochastic annealing scheme should lead us to the desired optimal point. It is very difficult, however, to give any guidance regarding good updating rules for β, and proper stopping criteria for the Markov chains. There are many general theoretical results available, but each specific problem requires its own fine tuning and there will always be a certain amount of trial and error involved.

11.3 Practical implementation issues

As soon as an MCMC algorithm suitable for the problem at hand has been determined, practical questions like the determination of starting points, burn-in periods and sample sizes have to be addressed. Here we briefly discuss these issues. The problem of estimating the expectation $E[f(X)]$, for some random variable X on E and some function f, by calculating time averages will serve as the main example throughout this section.

Starting point

First of all, we need a starting point for the Markov chain. A rapidly mixing chain will quickly find its way no matter how the starting value is chosen. On the other hand, some chains converge to stationarity very slowly unless the starting point is chosen carefully. If several processors are available on the computer it is always a good idea to run chains in parallel, all of them starting at different values.

Burn-in period

In order to reduce the risk of inferential bias caused by the effect of starting values, iterates during a certain initial period are usually discarded. The length of this burn-in period depends on the rate at which the Markov chain converges to stationarity. Ideally, we would like to compute this convergence rate, and use it to estimate the number of iteration steps needed. This is usually not a tractable problem: the power of MCMC methods lies in their ability to solve extremely complicated statistical problems, and complex MCMC solutions typically involve chains that are very difficult to analyse theoretically.

It is preferable to use *convergence diagnostics* (for a review, see Cowles and Carlin, 1994). Many different convergence diagnostics have been proposed in the literature, but they all have a common characteristic, namely that the sampler output is used in some way. Indeed, in many cases the output makes it obvious from the output when the initial transient period is over. We conclude by giving a simple rule of thumb that could be appropriate in some situations. If we are interested in estimating $E[f(X)]$ by computing time averages, then Geyer (1992) argues that since the burn-in period is likely to be less than 1% of the number of iterations needed to obtain adequate precision in the time average, we should concentrate on calculating the total run length needed and then just discard 1% of the iterations.

Sample size

How many iterations should we perform to ensure that our estimator is accurate enough? This question is also difficult to answer, because of the possible dependencies in the sample. We propose here some simple ideas that can be useful in particular circumstances.

First, if the iterates X_ν are indeed independent, then (assuming stationarity) the standard deviation of the time average $\sum_{\nu=1}^{n} f(X_\nu)/n$ is given by $\sigma/\sqrt{n}$, where σ is the standard deviation of $f(X)$. Alternatively, if the series can be approximated by a first order autoregressive process then the theory of time series tells us that the standard deviation of the time average is

$$\frac{\sigma}{\sqrt{n}}\sqrt{\frac{1+\rho}{1-\rho}},$$

where ρ is the autocorrelation of the series $f(X_\nu)$, and σ the standard deviation as above.

Another simple device used is to *thin* the observations by saving only every kth value, thus ensuring that the resulting sequence will consist of more or less independent values. In that case the simple sample mean $\sigma\sqrt{k/n}$ will again do the job. Finally, an obvious *ad hoc* method for determining the required run length is to run several chains in parallel, all with different starting points, and compare the resulting time averages. We shall not be satisfied until all of them agree adequately.

11.4 Bayesian inference for epidemics

In this final section we indicate why the development of MCMC methods has had such a profound effect on applied Bayesian statistics. Then, following O'Neill and Roberts (1999), we use MCMC to draw inferences on the infection probability when the final sizes of several household epidemics of Reed-Frost type are observed. We have deliberately chosen a very simple example, just to introduce the reader to the subject. The main topic in O'Neill and Roberts (1999) is inference on the infection and removal rates in the Markovian standard SIR epidemic model, after having observed the removal times. This investigation is also carried out using Markov Chain Monte Carlo in a Bayesian framework. Similar results can be achieved using other methods, see Becker and Hasofer (1997), but as soon as the models become slightly more complicated, e.g. by the introduction of latent periods, the flexibility in the MCMC approach becomes apparent.

From a Bayesian perspective, there is no real difference between observables and parameters of a statistical model: all are considered random quantities. Let D denote the observed data, and collect the model parameters and the missing data in a vector x. Then set up the joint distribution $p(D, x)$ over all random quantities. This distribution can be written

$$p(D, x) = p(x)L(D \mid x),$$

where $p(x)$ is the *prior* distribution of x and $L(D \mid x)$ is the *likelihood.* Bayes' theorem is now used to determine the *posterior* distribution of x given the observed data:

$$p(x \mid D) = \frac{p(x)L(D \mid x)}{\int p(y)L(D \mid y)\, dy}.$$

This posterior distribution is the object of all Bayesian inference.

The integral in the formula for $p(x \mid D)$ above is in general very difficult to compute, especially in high dimensions. However, by using the Metropolis-Hastings algorithm for sampling from the target distribution $\pi(x) = p(x \mid D)$ this problem is overcome very elegantly, since, as already noted below Eq. (11.1), normalizing factors in this target distribution never need to be computed. This is the main reason why MCMC has become such an important tool in Bayesian statistics.

Turning to the epidemic application, consider a population consisting of a number of households, each of size three. Start with one infectious individual in each household and run independent Reed-Frost epidemics. Denote the avoidance probability by q, so that $1-q$ is the probability that a given infective infects a given susceptible household member. Now, for $j = 0, 1, 2$, let N_j denote the number of households in which an epidemic of final size j has occurred. Our task is to estimate the avoidance probability q given the data $D = (N_0, N_1, N_2)$.

Recall from Section 1.2 that, for a given household,

$$\mathbf{P}(Z=0) = q^2, \quad \mathbf{P}(Z=1) = 2(1-q)q^2, \quad \mathbf{P}(Z=2) = (1-q)^2 + 2(1-q)^2 q.$$

Note that the first term in $\mathbf{P}(Z=2)$ is the probability of having the entire household infected in one generation while the second term is the probability that it takes two generations to infect the household. Denoting by $\tilde{N}_2$ the (unobserved) number of two generation-epidemics in the population, it follows that the likelihood function for q can be written

$$\begin{aligned} L(q|D,\tilde{N}_2) &= C(q^2)^{N_0}(2(1-q)q^2)^{N_1}((1-q)^2)^{N_2-\tilde{N}_2}(2(1-q)^2 q)^{\tilde{N}_2} \\ &= C \cdot 2^{N_1+\tilde{N}_2} q^{2N_0+2N_1+\tilde{N}_2}(1-q)^{N_1+2N_2}. \end{aligned}$$

Readers familiar with basic Bayesian statistics will notice from this equation that if a Beta(α, δ) distribution is chosen as the prior distribution of q, then the posterior distribution is given by

$$p(q \mid D, \tilde{N}_2) \sim \text{Beta}(2N_0 + 2N_1 + \tilde{N}_2 + \alpha, N_1 + 2N_2 + \delta). \tag{11.3}$$

Also, since the household epidemics are assumed to be independent, we have that

$$p(\tilde{N}_2 \mid D, q) \sim \text{Bin}\left(N_2, \frac{2q}{2q+1}\right). \tag{11.4}$$

The Gibbs sampler of Section 11.1 can now be used to sample from the target distribution $\pi(q, \tilde{N}_2) = p(q, \tilde{N}_2 \mid D)$, since we have the expressions (11.3) and (11.4) for the corresponding conditional distributions. By introducing the extra variable $\tilde{N}_2$ we were able to write the likelihood function in a convenient form, but the actual $\tilde{N}_2$-values will probably be regarded as uninteresting and may therefore not be included in the sample output.

Exercises

11.1. Show that the acceptance probability is 1 for the Gibbs sampler.

11.2. Implement the Gibbs sampler described in Section 11.4, and estimate the avoidance probability q from the hypothetical data given in the Table 11.1 below. All households had 1 initially infective and 2 initially susceptible individuals.

Table 11.1. Household outbreaks

Final size	Number of households
0	39
1	26
2	35

12 Vaccination

Perhaps the most important practical reason for the statistical analysis of epidemics lies in its application to vaccination policy. In the present chapter we focus on this topic. More precisely we consider the following question: who and how many individuals should be vaccinated to prevent future epidemic outbreaks? In Section 12.1 we study this question for the standard SIR epidemic, and in Section 12.2 for endemic diseases, focusing on estimates and neglecting uncertainties. The chapter concludes with a section devoted to the estimation of the vaccine efficacy, which measures the reduction in susceptibility resulting from vaccination. In Sections 12.1 and 12.3 we make use of the multitype epidemic presented in Chapter 6, where the types consist of vaccinated and unvaccinated individuals.

12.1 Estimating vaccination policies based on one epidemic

Assume that the standard SIR epidemic $E_{n,m}(\lambda, I)$ is observed in a large community. If the epidemic was observed completely, we can estimate the basic reproduction number θ using methods presented in Section 9.2 (see also the exercises); if the final size was observed, we use the methods of Section 10.1. Suppose now that a vaccine is available which reduces the transmission rate between an infectious and a vaccinated individual to $\lambda(1-r)/n$. The corresponding rate for a susceptible individual is λ/n, so r is the relative reduction, which is assumed to be known (its estimation is treated separately in Section 12.3). The important case of a perfect vaccine giving 100% and life-long immunity corresponds to $r = 1$. Based on the data from one outbreak, we wish to find the proportion v_c of the susceptible population, the critical vaccination coverage, that has to be vaccinated to prevent future outbreaks.

We first answer the question assuming θ to be known. Suppose a proportion v is vaccinated, then the community consists of two types of individuals, unvaccinated and vaccinated, and the multitype model of Chapter 6 is relevant. Adopting the notation of Chapter 6, we have two types of individual, 1 and 2 (unvaccinated and vaccinated) with $\pi_1 = 1 - v$ and $\pi_2 = v$. The infection parameters satisfy $\lambda_{11} = \lambda_{21} = \lambda$, $\lambda_{12} = \lambda_{22} = \lambda(1-r)$ and $\iota_1 = \iota_2 = \iota$; we are implicitly assuming that vaccination only reduces the risk of becoming infected and not the infectivity once infected. The reproduction number, here denoted by R_v for obvious reasons, is then according to Section 6.2 the largest eigenvalue of the matrix with coefficients $\{\iota_i\lambda_{ij}\pi_j\}$. For our specific case this eigenvalue is simply

$$R_v = \iota\lambda(1-v) + \iota\lambda(1-r)v. \tag{12.1}$$

From Section 6.2 we know that a major outbreak is impossible if $R_v \leq 1$. In terms of the proportion vaccinated v, this is equivalent to $v \geq (1 - 1/\theta)/r$ (remember that $\theta = \lambda\iota$ – the reproduction number prior to vaccination). This means that the critical

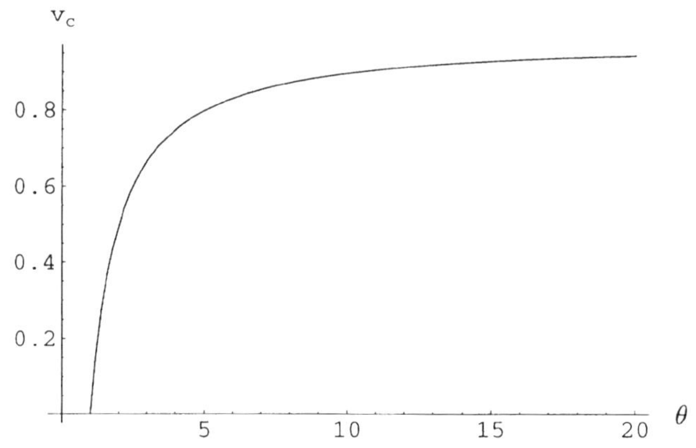

Figure 12.1: Graph of the critical vaccination coverage v_c plotted against θ.

vaccination (or immunity) coverage v_c, above which the population is protected from major outbreaks, is

$$v_c = \frac{1}{r}\left(1 - \frac{1}{\theta}\right).$$

It may happen that $v_c > 1$ (if r is small and θ large). The interpretation in this case is that the community is not protected from major outbreaks even when the whole community is vaccinated. The case with a perfect vaccine ($r = 1$) reduces to $v_c = 1 - 1/\theta$. The situation where the whole community, and not only vaccinated individuals, is protected from the epidemic is known as *herd immunity*. In Figure 12.1 above v_c is plotted against the basic reproduction number θ for the case of a perfect vaccine (i.e. $r = 1$). For example, if θ is known to equal 5, as may be the case for influenza, then the critical vaccination coverage is $v_c = 1 - 1/5 = 0.8$ which means that at least 80% of the community should be vaccinated in order to prevent an outbreak.

We now consider the case where θ is unknown. We then estimate it from observation of one epidemic outbreak (prior to vaccination) using theory from Chapter 9 or 10 depending on whether the epidemic is observed completely or only its final state is observed. Either way we get an estimate $\hat{\theta}$ (in case of complete data $\hat{\theta} = \hat{\lambda}\hat{\gamma}^{-1}$). We obviously estimate v_c by

$$\hat{v}_c = \frac{1}{r}\left(1 - \frac{1}{\hat{\theta}}\right). \tag{12.2}$$

Using the δ-method, we obtain the consistent standard error s.e.$(\hat{v}_c)$ = s.e.$(\hat{\theta})/r\hat{\theta}^2$. The standard error s.e.$(\hat{\theta})$ depends on the type of data. For final size data it is given in Corollary 10.2; for complete data it equals $\left((\hat{\gamma}^{-1} \times \text{s.e.}(\hat{\lambda}))^2 + (\hat{\lambda} \times \text{s.e.}(\hat{\gamma}^{-1}))^2\right)^{1/2}$, applying the δ-method and the fact that the two parameter estimates are independent. A confidence interval for v_c is obtained using the estimate and the standard error, together with the asymptotic normality of the estimator. Here it is most natural to use a one-sided confidence interval, since under-estimation has worse consequences than over-estimation.

In a heterogeneous community, the question of vaccination is more complex: now the effect of vaccination depends not only on the number vaccinated, but also on how individuals to be vaccinated are allocated. Suppose, for example, that the population consists of homogeneous individuals belonging to households where it is assumed that individuals mix at a higher rate within households, as in the model of Section 6.3. A relevant question is then how to select individuals for vaccination optimally, in the sense of most reducing the reproduction number. Is it better to spread vaccination over households or should one try to vaccinate certain households completely? Ball *et al.* (1997) show that for a sub-class of the model in Section 6.3 the optimal vaccination strategy is the 'equalizing' strategy. This strategy picks individuals sequentially from households with the largest number of remaining susceptible individuals, thus equalizing the number of remaining susceptibles in households. They conjecture this strategy to be optimal for the model in general. If instead the population is heterogeneous due to individual heterogeneities, such as varying infectivity and susceptibility, the same question of who to vaccinate is relevant. In case of equal infectivity one should vaccinate individuals with the highest susceptibility, but if the infectivity also varies there is no simple solution. Then there is a trade-off between high susceptibility and high infectivity in the optimal selection procedure.

The following important general question concerning estimation and vaccination was posed by Becker (e.g. Becker and Utev, 1998). Suppose an epidemic outbreak was observed and we want to draw inferences on who and how many to vaccinate. For a given model a vaccination strategy can often be derived, as with the standard SIR epidemic above. The question is how vaccination strategies derived from different model assumptions are related. That is, if a vaccination strategy was derived under the assumption that the observed epidemic was from model A, say, but model B is the true model, is the community still under herd immunity?

As an example, suppose 60% in a large, completely susceptible, community was infected during the epidemic season. With previous terminology we have $\bar{Z} = 0.6$ and we may assume that $\mu = 0$ (i.e. there were only few initial infectives). Assuming the epidemic is the standard SIR epidemic we can apply results from Chapter 10 to estimate $R_0 = \theta$ by $\hat{\theta} \approx -\ln(1-\bar{Z})/\bar{Z} = 1.53$. The critical vaccination coverage for a vaccine resulting in 90% reduction of susceptibility ($r = 0.9$) is then estimated from (12.2) as $\hat{v}_c = 0.9^{-1}(1 - 1.53^{-1}) = 0.384$. This means that at least 38.4% should be vaccinated for the community to possess herd immunity. A relevant question is whether the community possesses herd immunity if a random sample of the community of this size is vaccinated, when the model assumptions are false. Suppose that the community consisted of households, all of size four to keep things simple, and that the rate of transmission is higher within households. Is the community then protected from future outbreaks? Or suppose that in fact 40% of the females and 80% of the males were infected (implying that males are more susceptible). Is the community then under herd immunity? The answer to the first question for this specific example is 'yes', and to the second question 'no'.

There is no general answer for the first type of question, i.e. whether neglecting the presence of households, can result in under-estimation of the critical vaccination coverage. Becker and Utev (1998) show that if all households are of equal size then the critical vaccination coverage is lower than if the data was collected from a homogeneous community without households. However, if households are of different sizes, as in real life, then the relation can go either way (the direction depends on the household structure and the proportion infected). If the critical vaccination coverage is derived taking account of individual heterogeneities (men and women in the example above) then this proportion is *always* larger than the vaccination coverage derived neglecting heterogeneities (Britton, 1998b).

The natural conclusion is, of course, that heterogeneities should be taken into account. When doing this, one can also devise better vaccination strategies than picking individuals at random. The question is still important because it is reasonable to believe that some heterogeneities, social and/or individual, are not observable and therefore not taken into account. The results mentioned above then state that outbreaks may in fact occur in the community even when the proportion vaccinated exceeds v_c, if v_c is derived neglecting some relevant heterogeneities.

12.2 Estimating vaccination policies for endemic diseases

The question of who and how many individuals to vaccinate is perhaps even more important for endemic diseases. The prime example of an endemic infectious disease which has been completely eradicated by vaccination is smallpox. Presently most childhood diseases are subject to vaccination policies in the western world, and these diseases are no longer endemic in most parts. It is not possible to vaccinate everyone for practical and ethical reasons (e.g. some religious communities oppose vaccination). To derive the necessary proportion v_c to vaccinate (the critical vaccination coverage) is hence of great importance.

Below, we derive estimates for the two endemic models presented in Chapter 8. Because of the rather complicated structure of these models we shall not derive standard errors but only estimates. Of course, the models are over-simplified in that the community is assumed to be homogeneous and individuals are assumed to mix uniformly. Further, any seasonal effects are neglected, even though it is well-known that the beginning of school in the autumn usually implies outbreak peaks. Effects of vaccination policies, and their various estimation problems, for more realistic but deterministic models have been studied in many papers (e.g. Anderson and May, 1991, and Greenhalgh and Dietz, 1994).

The SIR model with demography

Let us first consider the SIR model with demography of Section 8.1, which we recapitulate briefly. New individuals are born at rate θn, an infectious individual has close contact with other individuals at rate λ (any specific individual at rate λ/n) and becomes removed at rate γ. Finally, each individual dies at rate θ irrespective of her disease state. The bivariate Markov process $(X, Y) = \{(X(t), Y(t)); t \geq 0\}$, which keeps track of the number of susceptibles and infectives respectively, is specified by the starting point $(n, \mu n)$ and its transition rates given in Section 8.1. Suppose now that a perfect vaccine is available, i.e. a vaccine giving life-long 100% immunity, and that a proportion v of all individuals are vaccinated at birth. The only transition rate that is affected is that susceptibles are born at rate $\theta(1-v)n$ (the remaining newborns are vaccinated and immune). We can apply the same model and results, with slight changes in the parameters as follows. Let $n' = n(1-v)$ so that susceptibles are born at rate $\theta n'$. For the jump rates to be consistent with the rates of Section 8.1, we then have to write n' in the transition rate for new infections, and this can be done if we introduce $\lambda' = \lambda(1-v)$. Thus, we have the model of Section 8.1 with n' and λ' replacing n and λ. Consequently the reproduction number R_v after the vaccination scheme is started, is given by

$$R_v = \frac{\lambda'}{\gamma+\theta} = \frac{\lambda(1-v)}{\gamma+\theta} = (1-v)R_0.$$

From properties of the model it then follows that the only stationary point is the disease-free state if $R_v < 1$. This is equivalent to $v > 1 - 1/R_0$. The critical vaccination coverage is hence

$$v_c = 1 - \frac{1}{R_0} = 1 - \frac{\gamma+\theta}{\lambda}.$$

If R_0 is unknown it may be estimated prior to vaccination by observing the community in its stationary state. From Section 8.1 we know that in case of endemicity, the stationary point for population proportions is given by $(\hat{x}, \hat{y}) = \left(R_0^{-1}, (R_0-1)(\alpha R_0)^{-1}\right)$. From this it immediately follows that R_0 is estimated by the inverse of x_{obs}, the observed proportion of susceptibles: $\hat{R}_0 = 1/x_{obs}$. To conclude, an estimate of the critical vaccination coverage v_c necessary to prevent future outbreaks is

$$\hat{v}_c = 1 - x_{obs}. \tag{12.3}$$

Consider as an example measles in the western world prior to vaccination. On the average a fraction of approximately $1/15 \approx 7\%$ had not yet experienced the disease and were thus susceptible. This implies that $\hat{v}_c \approx 93\%$, and a vaccination coverage above this value will eradicate the disease. The vaccination coverage of measles in the United States has by now exceeded 90% and the disease is no longer endemic - only smaller local outbreaks still occur. This shows that the estimate is in the right ball park even though it is estimated from a simple model neglecting heterogeneities in the community as well as social and geographic structure.

Because most individuals will experience the disease before dying, and all individuals live equally long on the average, the community proportion of susceptibles will coincide with the average fraction of an individual's life that she is susceptible. That is, the average age at infection divided by the average lifetime. Conversely, the average age of infection is the average lifetime divided by R_0. This explains the name 'childhood disease': the (average) age of infection is small mainly because R_0 is large, and not because of the special behaviour of children. For example, measles is believed to have $R_0 \approx 15$, so with an average lifetime of 75 years the formula states that the average age at infection is 75/15=5 years.

The SIS model

In the SIS model (Section 8.2), the community is fixed and new susceptibles arise not from births of new individuals but from infectious individuals recovering and becoming susceptible (in SIR models they become immune after recovery or die). An infectious individual has close contact with others at rate λ (λ/n with any specific individual) and an infectious individual recovers and becomes susceptible at rate γ. The transition rates for the induced Markov process are given in Section 8.2 where properties of the model are also presented. The basic reproduction number satisfies $R_0 = \lambda/\gamma$ and the epidemic dies out quickly unless $R_0 > 1$. Assume as in the previous paragraph that a perfect vaccine is available and that the proportion v of all individuals is vaccinated. This affects the transition rate corresponding to infection: if there are i infectives the number of susceptibles is $n(1-v)-i$ (and not $n-i$ as it is prior to vaccination). However, if we replace n by $n' = n(1-v)$ and λ by $\lambda' = \lambda(1-v)$ the transition rates for the vaccinated community coincide with the rates of Section 8.2. From results of Section 8.2 it thus follows that the epidemic will surely become extinct if $\lambda'/\gamma \le 1$, which is equivalent to $v \ge 1-\gamma/\lambda$. The critical vaccination coverage is therefore

$$v_c = 1 - \frac{\gamma}{\lambda} = 1 - \frac{1}{R_0}.$$

Prior to vaccination the proportion of susceptibles converges to $\gamma/\lambda = 1/R_0$. If R_0 is unknown it can hence be estimated by the inverse of x_{obs}, the observed proportion of susceptibles for a community in its stationary state. An estimate for the critical vaccination coverage is thus

$$\hat{v}_c = 1 - x_{obs}.$$

We see that this is the same estimate as in the SIR model with demography (12.3). The relation $v_c = 1 - 1/R_0$ holds for a larger class of models including the models assuming homogeneous mixing and a homogeneous community.

12.3 Estimation of vaccine efficacy

We now proceed to estimate the parameter r defined in Section 12.1 as the relative reduction in the rate at which vaccinated individuals become infected by infectious individuals, compared with the rate for unvaccinated individuals (the rate for unvaccinated is λ/n and $\lambda(1-r)/n$ for vaccinated). It is assumed that the infectivity of vaccinated individuals is unchanged. That is, if a vaccinated individual becomes infected she is infectious as she would have been if not vaccinated. We estimate r assuming that we observe the standard SIR epidemic in which part of the community is vaccinated and the rest are not. To keep things simple we assume a large community in which a negligible fraction is vaccinated. Alternative methods for estimating r can be derived from a matched pair study, for example with sibling pairs where one sibling is vaccinated and the other is not.

Assume that a sample of size ν among the n susceptibles ($\pi_v = \nu/n$ being negligible) were selected and vaccinated prior to the epidemic. After the epidemic outbreak has run its course, a proportion $\bar{Z}_u$ of the unvaccinated and a proportion $\bar{Z}_v$ of the vaccinated are found to have been infected. The initial proportion of infectives is assumed to be small. The overall proportion infected is $\bar{Z} = \pi_v \bar{Z}_v + (1-\pi_v)\bar{Z}_u \approx \bar{Z}_u$. According to Section 6.2, in case of a major outbreak $(\bar{Z}_u, \bar{Z}_v)$ converges in probability to (τ_u, τ_v), the positive solution of

$$\begin{aligned} 1-\tau_u &= e^{-\iota\lambda(\pi_v\tau_v+(1-\pi_v)\tau_u)} \\ 1-\tau_v &= e^{-(1-r)\iota\lambda(\pi_v\tau_v+(1-\pi_v)\tau_u)}. \end{aligned}$$

From these equations it follows that $1 - r = \log(1-\tau_v)/\log(1-\tau_u)$. Replacing the limiting quantities by the corresponding observed values gives an estimate of r:

$$\hat{r} = 1 - \frac{\log(1-\bar{Z}_v)}{\log(1-\bar{Z}_u)}. \tag{12.4}$$

Up until now, we have not made use of the assumption that the proportion vaccinated π_v is small, and consequently the estimate is consistent without this assumption. A standard error for the estimate can also be derived for the general case using the central limit theorem of Ball and Clancy (1993) presented in Section 6.2. Here we treat the simpler case with π_v assumed to be small. This implies that $\bar{Z}_u$ can be treated as deterministic in comparison with $\bar{Z}_v$. Because the proportion vaccinated is negligible these individuals do not affect the overall proportion infected. Thus, each vaccinated individual behaves more or less independently and becomes infected with probability $\tau_v = 1 - e^{-(1-r)\iota\lambda(\pi_v\tau_v+(1-\pi_v)\tau_u)}$. Consequently Z_v is binomially distributed with parameters ν and τ_v. Treating $\bar{Z}_u$ as deterministic, we see from equation (12.4) that the variance of $\hat{r}$ equals the variance of $\log(1-\bar{Z}_v)$ divided by $(\log(1-\bar{Z}_u))^2$. Expanding $\log(1-\bar{Z}_v)$ in a Taylor series, and applying the δ-method it follows that the variance of $\log(1-\bar{Z}_v)$ approximately equals the variance of $\bar{Z}_v$ divided by $(1-\tau_v)^2$. Finally, the variance of $\bar{Z}_v$ is $\tau_v(1-\tau_v)/\nu$ since Z_v is binomially distributed, and this may be estimated by $\bar{Z}_v(1-\bar{Z}_v)/\nu$. A consistent estimate of the standard deviation of $\hat{r}$ is thus

$$\text{s.e.}(\hat{r}) = \frac{\sqrt{\bar{Z}_v(1-\bar{Z}_v)}}{\sqrt{\nu}(1-\bar{Z}_v)|\log(1-\bar{Z}_u)|}. \tag{12.5}$$

As an example, suppose that in a large community 50% of the unvaccinated were infected while only 10% in the sample of $\nu = 200$ vaccinated individuals were infected. This means $\bar{Z}_u = 0.5$ and $\bar{Z}_v = 0.1$. Equations (12.4) then gives $\hat{r} = 0.848$ and $\text{s.e.}(\hat{r}) = 0.034$ from (12.5).

The parameter r measures the reduction in transmission which is a natural measure of the efficacy of a vaccine. Traditionally however, the definition of the vaccine efficacy VE is

$$VE = 1 - \frac{\bar{Z}_v}{\bar{Z}_u},$$

using the terminology of the present section. This measure is not a very satisfactory single measure of the vaccine efficacy because it depends on the proportion vaccinated and on the community from which data come. That is, one would get a different estimate if a larger/smaller proportion were vaccinated prior to the epidemic, and also in a different community in which individuals mix at higher/lower rate. The parameter r is to be preferred, as it does not have these unsatisfactory properties.

Exercises

12.1. Check that the formula for R_v, given in equation (12.1), actually gives the largest eigenvalue to the specified matrix.

12.2. As discussed in the introduction of Part II and in Exercise 9.4 the estimates of Part II can be modified to cover the case with initially immune individuals (for simplicity the text is written assuming no initially immune individuals). Suppose the proportion initially infectious is negligible ($\mu \approx 0$) and that s is the initial proportion susceptible. Then it is not hard to show (simply by transforming parameters) that the ultimate proportion infected *among the initially susceptibles* converges in probability to a solution of the equation $1 - e^{\theta s \tau}$ to be compared with equation (4.2) for the case with no initially immunes (remember that $\theta = \lambda\iota$). This implies that the estimates of the present section are not estimates of θ but of θs. Derive estimates and confidence bounds for θ and v_c assuming that the initial proportion susceptible s is known and where data consists of knowing the observed proportion infected among those initially suceptible.

12.3. Estimate and derive standard error for the critical vaccination coverage v_c for the smallpox outbreak presented in Exercise 9.3.

a) assuming complete data.

b) assuming that only the final state is observed (see Exercise 10.1).

12.4. Estimate v_c for the Tristan da Cunha outbreak presented in Exercise 10.2.

12.5. Suppose that 10 years is the average age at infection of some childhood disease in a society with average life-length of 70 years. Assume that the SIR model with demography applies and derive an estimate of v_c, the proportion necessary to vaccinate to surely prevent future outbreaks.

12.6. Suppose a hypothetical vaccine trial resulted in 16 infected individuals among the sample of 185 vaccinated individuals whereas 42% of the remaining (large number of) individuals were infected. Derive an estimate of the reduction parameter r and give a standard error for the estimate.

References

Addy C. L., Longini I. M. and Haber M. (1991): A generalized stochastic model for the analysis of infectious disease final size data. *Biometrics* **47**, 961-974.

Aldous D. (1989): *Probability approximations via the Poisson clumping heuristics.* Springer-Verlag, New York.

Altmann M. (1995): Susceptible-Infected-Removed epidemic models with dynamic partnerships. *J. Math. Biol.* **33**, 661-675.

Altmann M. (1998): The deterministic limit of infectious disease models with dynamic partners. *Math. Biosci.,* **150**, 153-175.

Andersen P. K., Borgan Ø., Gill R. D. and Keiding N. (1993): *Statistical models based on counting processes.* Springer, New York.

Anderson R. M. and May R. M. (1991): *Infectious diseases of humans; dynamics and control.* Oxford University Press, Oxford.

Andersson H. (1998): Limit theorems for a random graph epidemic model. *Ann. Appl. Prob.* **8**, 1331-1349.

Andersson H. (2000): Epidemic models on social networks. To appear in The Mathematical Scientist.

Andersson H. and Britton T. (1998): Heterogeneity in epidemic models and its effect on the spread of infection. *J. Appl. Prob.* **35**, 651-661.

Andersson H. and Djehiche B. (1998): A threshold limit theorem for the stochastic logistic epidemic. *J. Appl. Prob.* **35**, 662-670.

von Bahr B. and Martin-Löf A. (1980): Threshold limit theorems for some epidemic processes. *Adv. Appl. Prob.* **12**, 319-349.

Bailey N. T. J. (1953): The total size of a general stochastic epidemic. *Biometrika* **40**, 177-185.

Bailey N. T. J. (1975): *The mathematical theory of infectious diseases and its applications.* Griffin, London.

Ball F. (1985): Deterministic and stochastic epidemics with several kinds of susceptibles. *Adv. Appl. Prob.* **17**, 1-22.

Ball F. (1986): A unified approch to the distribution of total size and total area under the trajectory of infectives in epidemic models. *Adv. Appl. Prob.* **18**, 289-310.

Ball F. (1995): Coupling methods in epidemic theory, in *Epidemic models: Their structure and relation to data.* Mollison D., Ed., Publications of the Newton Institute, Cambridge University Press, Cambridge.

Ball F. and Barbour A. D. (1990): Poisson approximation for some epidemic models. *J. Appl. Prob.* **27**, 479-490.

Ball F. and Clancy D. (1993): The final size and severity of a generalised stochastic multitype epidemic model. *Adv. Appl. Prob.* **25**, 721-736.

Ball F. and Donnelly P. (1995): Strong approximations for epidemic models. *Stoch. Proc. Appl.* **55**, 1-21.

Ball F., Mollison D. and Scalia-Tomba G. (1997): Epidemics with two levels of mixing. *Ann. Appl. Prob.* **7**, 46-89.

Barbour A. D. (1975): The duration of the closed stochastic epidemic. *Biometrika* **62**, 477-482.

Barbour A. D., Lindvall T. and Rogers L. C. G. (1991): Stochastic ordering of order statistics. *J. Appl. Prob.* **28**, 278-286.

Barbour A. D., Holst L. and Janson S. (1992): *Poisson approximation.* Oxford University Press, Oxford.

Barbour A. D. and Mollison D. (1990): Epidemics and random graphs, in *Stochastic processes in epidemic theory.* Gabriel J. P., Lefèvre C. and Picard P., Eds., *Lecture notes in Biomathematics* **86**, 86-89.

Bartlett M. S. (1949): Some evolutionary stochastic processes. *J. Roy. Statist. Soc. B* **11**, 211-229.

Bartlett M. S. (1955): *An introduction to stochastic processes.* Cambridge University Press, Cambridge.

Bartlett M. S. (1956): Deterministic and stochastic models for recurrent epidemics. *Proc. Third Berkeley Symp. Math. Statist, & Prob.* **4**, 81-109. Univ. California Press, Berkeley and Los Angeles.

Bartoszyński R. (1972): On a certain model of an epidemic. *Applicationes Mathematicae* **13**, 139-151.

Becker N. G. (1989): *Analysis of Infectious Disease Data.* Chapman and Hall, London.

Becker N. G. (1997): Uses of the EM algorithm in the analysis of data on HIV/AIDS and other infectious diseases. *Statist. Meth. Med. Research* **6**, in press.

Becker N. G. and Britton T. (1999): Statistical studies of infectious disease incidence. *J. Roy. Statist. Soc. B,* **61**, 287-307.

Becker N. G. and Dietz K. (1995): The effect of the household distribution on transmission and control of highly infectious diseases. *Math. Biosci.* **127**, 207-219.

Becker N. G. and Hall R. (1996): Immunization levels for preventing epidemics in a community of households made up of individuals of different types. *Math. Biosci.* **132**, 205-216.

Becker N. G. and Hasofer A. M. (1997): Estimation in epidemics with incomplete observations. *J. Roy. Statist. Soc. B,***59**, 415-429.

Becker N. G. and Starczak D. N. (1997): Optimal vaccination strategies for a community of households. *Math. Biosci.* **129**, 117-132.

Becker N. G. and Utev S. (1998): The effect of community structure on the immunity coverage required to prevent epidemics. *Math Biosci,* **147**, 23-39.

Billingsley P. (1968): *Convergence of probability measures.* Wiley, New York.

Bollobás B. (1985): *Random graphs.* Academic Press, New York.

Britton T. (1998a): Estimation in multitype epidemics. *J. Roy. Statist. Soc. B,* **60**, 663-679.

Britton T. (1998b): On the critical vaccination coverage in multitype epidemics. *J. Appl. Prob.,* **35** 1003-1006.

Cox D. R. (1972): Regression models and life tables (with discussion). *J. Roy. Statist. Soc. B* **34**, 187-220.

Cox J. T. and Durrett R. (1988): Limit theorems for the spread of epidemics and forest fires. *Stoch. Proc. Appl.* **30**, 171-191.

Daley D. J. and Gani J. (1999): *Epidemic Modelling: an introduction.* Cambridge University Press, Cambdridge.

Daley D. J. and Kendall D. G. (1965): Stochastic rumours. *J. Inst. Maths. Applics.* **1**, 42-55.

Dempster A. P., Laird N. M. and Rubin D. B. (1977): Maximum Likelihood from incomplete data via the *EM* algorithm (with Discussion) J. Roy. Statist. Soc. B, **39**, 1-38.

Diekmann O. and Heesterbeek J.A.P. (200?): *Mathematical Epidemiology of Infectious Diseases: Model Building, Analysis and Interpretation.* (In preparation.) Wiley Series in Mathematical and Computational Biology.

Diekmann O., de Jong M. C. M. and Metz J. A. J (1998): A deterministic epidemic model taking account of repeated contacts between the same individuals. *J. Appl. Prob.* **35**, 448-462.

van Doorn E. A. (1991): Quasi-stationary distributions and convergence to quasi-stationarity of birth-death processes. *Adv. Appl. Prob.* **23**, 683-700.

Durrett R. (1995): Ten lectures on particle systems. *Springer Lecture Notes in Math.* **1608**, 97-201.

Erdős P. and Rényi A. (1959): On random graphs I. *Publ. Math. Debrecen* **6**, 290-297.

Ethier S. N. and Kurtz T. G. (1986): *Markov Processes: Characterization and Convergence.* Wiley, New York.

Gabriel J.-P., Lefèvre C. and Picard P. (Eds.) (1990): *Stochastic Processes in Epidemic Theory.* Springer Lecture Notes in Biomath, **86**.

Geyer C. J. (1992): Practical Markov chain Monte Carlo. *Statist. Sci.* **7**, 473-511.

Gilks W. R., Richardson S. and Spiegelhalter D. J. (1996): *Markov Chain Monte Carlo in practice.* Chapman & Hall, London.

Gontcharoff W. (1937): *Détermination des fonctions entières par interpolation.* Hermann, Paris.

Greenhalgh D. and Dietz K. (1994): Some bounds on estimates for reproduction ratio derived from the age-specific force of infection. *Math. Biosci.* **124**, 9-57.

Grenfell B. and Dobson A. (1995): *Ecology of infectious diseases in natural populations.* Cambridge University Press, Cambridge.

Hamer W. H. (1906): The Milroy lectures on epidemic disease in England – the evidence of variability and persistence of type. *The Lancet* **1**, 733-739.

van Herwaarden O. A. and Grasman J. (1995): Stochastic epidemics: major outbreaks and the duration of the endemic period. *J. Math. Biol.* **33**, 581-601.

Hougaard P. (1995): Frailty models for survival data. *Lifetime data analysis* **1**, 255-273.

Isham V. and Medley G. (1996): *Models for infectious human diseases: Their structure and relation to data.* Cambridge University Press, Cambridge.

Islam M. N., O'Shaughnessy C. D. and Smith B. (1996): A random graph model for the final-size distribution of household infections. *Statistics in Medicine* **15**, 837-843.

Jagers P. (1975): *Branching processes with biological applications.* Wiley, London.

Karatzas I. and Shreve S. E. (1991): *Brownian motion and stochastic calculus.* 2nd edn., Springer-Verlag, New York.

Keilson J. (1979): *Markov Chain Models–Rarity and Exponentiality.* Springer-Verlag, New York.

Kendall D. (1956): Deterministic and stochastic epidemics in closed populations, in *Proc. 3rd Berkeley Symp. Math. Statist. Prob.* **4**, 149-165.

Kermack W. O. and McKendrick A. G. (1927): A contribution to the mathematical theory of epidemics. *Proc. Roy. Soc. Lond. A* **115**, 700-721.

Kesten H. (1982): *Percolation theory for mathematicians.* Birkhauser, Boston.

Kurtz T. G. (1981): *Approximations of Population Processes. CBMS-NSF Regional Conf. Series in Appl. Math.* **36**, SIAM, Philadelphia.

Kuulasmaa K. (1982): The spatial general epidemic and locally dependent random graphs. *J. Appl. Prob.* **19**, 745-758.

Kuulasmaa K. and Zachary S. (1984): On spatial general epidemics and bond percolation processes. *J. Appl. Prob.* **21**, 911-914.

Lefèvre C. and Picard P. (1990): A non-standard family of polynomials and the final size distribution of Reed-Frost epidemic processes. *Adv. Appl. Prob.* **22**, 25-48.

Liggett T. M. (1985): *Interacting particle systems.* Springer, New York.

Lindvall T. (1992): *Lectures on the coupling method.* Wiley, New York.

Longini I. M. and Koopman J. S. (1982): Household and community transmission parameters from final distributions of infections in households. *Biometrics* **38**, 115-126.

Ludwig D. (1974): Stochastic population theories. *Lecture notes in Biomathematics* **3**.

Maki D. P. and Thompson M. (1973): *Mathematical models and applications*. Prentice-Hall, Englewood Cliffs, NJ.

McKendrick A. G. (1926): Applications of mathematics to medical problems. *Proc. Edinburgh Math. Soc.* **14**, 98-130.

Metropolis N., Rosenblutt A. W., Rosenblutt M. N., Teller A. H., Teller E. (1953): Equations of state calculations of fast computing machine. *J. Chem. Phys.* **21**, 1087-1091.

Mollison D. (1977): Spatial contact models for ecological and epidemic spread (with discussion). *J. Roy. Statist. Soc. B* **39**, 283-326.

Mollison D. (Ed.) (1995): *Epidemic Models: Their structure and relation to data.* Cambridge University Press, Cambridge.

Nåsell I. (1996): The quasi-stationary distribution of the closed endemic SIS model. *Adv. Appl. Prob.* **28**, 895-932.

Nåsell I. (1999): On the time to extinction in recurrent epidemics. *J. Roy. Statist. Soc. B.* **61**, 309-330.

O'Neill P., Balding D., Becker N., Eerola M. and Mollison D. (200?): Analyses of infectious disease data from household outbreaks by Markov Chain Monte Carlo methods. To appear in *Applied Statistics*.

O'Neill P. and Roberts G. (1999): Bayesian inference for partially observed stochastic epidemics. *J. Roy. Statist. Soc. A.***162**, 121-129.

Proschan F. and Sethuraman J. (1976): Stochastic comparison of order statistics from heterogeneous populations, with applications in reliability. *J. Multivariate Anal.* **6**, 608-616.

Rand D. A. (1997): Correlation equations and pair approximations for spatial ecologies, in *Theoretical Ecology 2*. McGlade J., Ed., Blackwell Scientific Publishing.

Rebolledo R. (1980): Central limit theorems for local martingales. *Z. Wahrsch. Verw. Gebiete.* **51**, 269-286.

Rhodes P. H., Halloran M. E. and Longini I. M. (1996): Counting process models for infectious disease data: distinguishing exposure to infection from susceptibility. *J.R. Statist. Soc. B,* **58**, 751-762.

Rida W. N. (1991): Asymptotic properties of some estimators for the infection rate in the general stochastic epidemic. *J.R. Statist. Soc. B,* **53**, 269-283.

Roberts G. O. and Smith A. F. M. (1994): Simple conditions for the convergence of the Gibbs sampler and Hastings-Metropolis algorithms. *Stoch. Proc. Appl.* **49**, 207-216.

Ross R. (1908): Report on the prevention of malaria in Mauritius. London.

Scalia-Tomba G. (1985): Asymptotic final size distribution for some chain-binomial processes. *Adv. Appl. Prob.* **17**, 477-495.

Scalia-Tomba G. (1990): On the asymptotic final size distribution of epidemics in heterogeneous populations, in *Stochastic processes in epidemic theory.* Gabriel J. P., Lefèvre C. and Picard P., Eds., *Lecture notes in Biomathematics* **86**, 189-196.

Sellke T. (1983): On the asymptotic distribution of the size of a stochastic epidemic. *J. Appl. Prob.* **20**, 390-394.

Syski R. (1992): *Passage times for Markov chains.* IOS Press, Amsterdam.

Whittle P. (1955): The outcome of a stochastic epidemic – a note on Bailey's paper, *Biometrika* **42**, 116-122.

Subject index

Lecture Notes in Statistics

For information about Volumes 1 to 77,
please contact Springer-Verlag

Vol. 78: L. Fahrmeir, B. Francis, R. Gilchrist, G. Tutz (Eds.), Advances in GLIM and Statistical Modelling: Proceedings of the GLIM92 Conference and the 7th International Workshop on Statistical Modelling, Munich, 13-17 July 1992. ix, 225 pages, 1992.

Vol. 79: N. Schmitz, Optimal Sequentially Planned Decision Procedures. xii, 209 pages, 1992.

Vol. 80: M. Fligner, J. Verducci (Eds.), Probability Models and Statistical Analyses for Ranking Data. xxii, 306 pages, 1992.

Vol. 81: P. Spirtes, C. Glymour, R. Scheines, Causation, Prediction, and Search. xxiii, 526 pages, 1993.

Vol. 82: A. Korostelev and A. Tsybakov, Minimax Theory of Image Reconstruction. xii, 268 pages, 1993.

Vol. 83: C. Gatsonis, J. Hodges, R. Kass, N. Singpurwalla (Editors), Case Studies in Bayesian Statistics. xii, 437 pages, 1993.

Vol. 84: S. Yamada, Pivotal Measures in Statistical Experiments and Sufficiency. vii, 129 pages, 1994.

Vol. 85: P. Doukhan, Mixing: Properties and Examples. xi, 142 pages, 1994.

Vol. 86: W. Vach, Logistic Regression with Missing Values in the Covariates. xi, 139 pages, 1994.

Vol. 87: J. Müller, Lectures on Random Voronoi Tessellations.vii, 134 pages, 1994.

Vol. 88: J. E. Kolassa, Series Approximation Methods in Statistics. Second Edition, ix, 183 pages, 1997.

Vol. 89: P. Cheeseman, R.W. Oldford (Editors), Selecting Models From Data: AI and Statistics IV. xii, 487 pages, 1994.

Vol. 90: A. Csenki, Dependability for Systems with a Partitioned State Space: Markov and Semi-Markov Theory and Computational Implementation. x, 241 pages, 1994.

Vol. 91: J.D. Malley, Statistical Applications of Jordan Algebras. viii, 101 pages, 1994.

Vol. 92: M. Eerola, Probabilistic Causality in Longitudinal Studies. vii, 133 pages, 1994.

Vol. 93: Bernard Van Cutsem (Editor), Classification and Dissimilarity Analysis. xiv, 238 pages, 1994.

Vol. 94: Jane F. Gentleman and G.A. Whitmore (Editors), Case Studies in Data Analysis. viii, 262 pages, 1994.

Vol. 95: Shelemyahu Zacks, Stochastic Visibility in Random Fields. x, 175 pages, 1994.

Vol. 96: Ibrahim Rahimov, Random Sums and Branching Stochastic Processes. viii, 195 pages, 1995.

Vol. 97: R. Szekli, Stochastic Ordering and Dependence in Applied Probability. viii, 194 pages, 1995.

Vol. 98: Philippe Barbe and Patrice Bertail, The Weighted Bootstrap. viii, 230 pages, 1995.

Vol. 99: C.C. Heyde (Editor), Branching Processes: Proceedings of the First World Congress. viii, 185 pages, 1995.

Vol. 100: Wlodzimierz Bryc, The Normal Distribution: Characterizations with Applications. viii, 139 pages, 1995.

Vol. 101: H.H. Andersen, M.Højbjerre, D. Sørensen, P.S.Eriksen, Linear and Graphical Models: for the Multivariate Complex Normal Distribution. x, 184 pages, 1995.

Vol. 102: A.M. Mathai, Serge B. Provost, Takesi Hayakawa, Bilinear Forms and Zonal Polynomials. x, 378 pages, 1995.

Vol. 103: Anestis Antoniadis and Georges Oppenheim (Editors), Wavelets and Statistics. vi, 411 pages, 1995.

Vol. 104: Gilg U.H. Seeber, Brian J. Francis, Reinhold Hatzinger, Gabriele Steckel-Berger (Editors), Statistical Modelling: 10th International Workshop, Innsbruck, July 10-14th 1995. x, 327 pages, 1995.

Vol. 105: Constantine Gatsonis, James S. Hodges, Robert E. Kass, Nozer D. Singpurwalla(Editors), Case Studies in Bayesian Statistics, Volume II. x, 354 pages, 1995.

Vol. 106: Harald Niederreiter, Peter Jau-Shyong Shiue (Editors), Monte Carlo and Quasi-Monte Carlo Methods in Scientific Computing. xiv, 372 pages, 1995.

Vol. 107: Masafumi Akahira, Kei Takeuchi, Non-Regular Statistical Estimation. vii, 183 pages, 1995.

Vol. 108: Wesley L. Schaible (Editor), Indirect Estimators in U.S. Federal Programs. viii, 195 pages, 1995.

Vol. 109: Helmut Rieder (Editor), Robust Statistics, Data Analysis, and Computer Intensive Methods. xiv, 427 pages, 1996.

Vol. 110: D. Bosq, Nonparametric Statistics for Stochastic Processes. xii, 169 pages, 1996.

Vol. 111: Leon Willenborg, Ton de Waal, Statistical Disclosure Control in Practice. xiv, 152 pages, 1996.

Vol. 112: Doug Fischer, Hans-J. Lenz (Editors), Learning from Data. xii, 450 pages, 1996.

Vol. 113: Rainer Schwabe, Optimum Designs for Multi-Factor Models. viii, 124 pages, 1996.

Vol. 114: C.C. Heyde, Yu. V. Prohorov, R. Pyke, and S. T. Rachev (Editors), Athens Conference on Applied Probability and Time Series Analysis Volume I: Applied Probability In Honor of J.M. Gani. viii, 424 pages, 1996.

Vol. 115: P.M. Robinson, M. Rosenblatt (Editors), Athens Conference on Applied Probability and Time Series Analysis Volume II: Time Series Analysis In Memory of E.J. Hannan. viii, 448 pages, 1996.

Vol. 116. Genshiro Kitagawa and Will Gersch, Smoothness Priors Analysis of Time Series. x, 261 pages, 1996.

Vol. 117: Paul Glasserman, Karl Sigman, David D. Yao (Editors), Stochastic Networks. xii, 298, 1996.

Vol. 118: Radford M. Neal, Bayesian Learning for Neural Networks. xv, 183, 1996.

Vol. 119. Masanao Aoki, Arthur M. Havenner, Applications of Computer Aided Time Series Modeling. ix, 329 pages, 1997.

Vol. 120: Maia Berkane, Latent Variable Modeling and Applications to Causality. vi, 288 pages, 1997.

Vol. 121: Constantine Gatsonis, James S. Hodges, Robert E. Kass, Robert McCulloch, Peter Rossi, Nozer D. Singpurwalla (Editors), Case Studies in Bayesian Statistics, Volume III. xvi, 487 pages, 1997.

Vol. 122. Timothy G. Gregoire, David R. Brillinger, Peter J. Diggle, Estelle Russek-Cohen, William G. Warren, Russell D. Wolfinger (Editors), Modeling Longitudinal and Spatially Correlated Data. x, 402 pages, 1997.

Vol. 123. D. Y. Lin and T. R. Fleming (Editors), Proceedings of the First Seattle Symposium in Biostatistics: Survival Analysis. xiii, 308 pages, 1997.

Vol. 124: Christine H. Muller, Robust Planning and Analysis of Experiments. x, 234 pages, 1997.

Vol. 125: Valerii V. Fedorov and Peter Hackl, Model-oriented Design of Experiments. viii, 117 pages, 1997.

Vol. 126: Geert Verbeke and Geert Molenberghs, Linear Mixed Models in Practice: A SAS-Oriented Approach. xiii, 306 pages, 1997.

Vol. 127. Harald Niederreiter, Peter Hellekalek, Gerhard Larcher, and Peter Zinterhof (Editors), Monte Carlo and Quasi-Monte Carlo Methods 1996, xii, 448 pages, 1997.

Vol. 128. L. Accardi and C.C. Heyde (Editors), Probability Towards 2000, x, 356 pages, 1998.

Vol. 129: Wolfgang Härdle, Gerard Kerkyacharian, Dominique Picard, and Alexander Tsybakov, Wavelets, Approximation, and Statistical Applications, xvi, 265 pages, 1998.

Vol. 130: Bo-Cheng Wei, Exponential Family Nonlinear Models, ix, 240 pages, 1998.

Vol. 131. Joel L. Horowitz, Semiparametric Methods in Econometrics, ix, 204 pages, 1998.

Vol. 132. Douglas Nychka, Walter W. Piegorsch, and Lawrence H. Cox (Editors), Case Studies in Environmental Statistics, viii, 200 pages, 1998.

Vol. 133: Dipak Dey, Peter Müller, and Debajyoti Sinha (Editors), Practical Nonparametric and Semiparametric Bayesian Statistics, xv, 408 pages, 1998.

Vol. 134: Yu. A. Kutoyants, Statistical Inference For Spatial Poisson Processes, vii, 284 pages, 1998.

Vol. 135: Christian P. Robert, Discretization and MCMC Convergence Assessment, x, 192 pages, 1998.

Vol. 136. Gregory C. Reinsel, Raja P. Velu, Multivariate Reduced-Rank Regression, xiii, 272 pages, 1998.

Vol. 137: V. Seshadri, The Inverse Gaussian Distribution: Statistical Theory and Applications, xi, 360 pages, 1998.

Vol. 138: Peter Hellekalek, Gerhard Larcher (Editors), Random and Quasi-Random Point Sets, xi, 352 pages, 1998.

Vol. 139. Roger B. Nelsen, An Introduction to Copulas, xi, 232 pages, 1999.

Vol. 140: Constantine Gatsonis, Robert E. Kass, Bradley Carlin, Alicia Carriquiry, Andrew Gelman, Isabella Verdinelli, Mike West (Editors), Case Studies in Bayesian Statistics, Volume IV, xvi, 456 pages, 1999.

Vol. 141: Peter Müller, Brani Vidakovic (Editors), Bayesian Inference in Wavelet Based Models, xi, 394 pages, 1999.

Vol. 142: György Terdik, Bilinear Stochastic Models and Related Problems of Nonlinear Time Series Analysis: A Frequency Domain Approach, xi, 258 pages, 1999.

Vol. 143: Russell Barton, Graphical Methods for the Design of Experiments, x, 208 pages, 1999.

Vol. 144: L. Mark Berliner, Douglas Nychka, and Timothy Hoar (Editors), Case Studies in Statistics and the Atmospheric Sciences, x, 208 pages, 1999.

Vol. 145. James H. Matis and Thomas R. Kiffe, Stochastic Population Models, viii, 220 pages, 2000.

Vol. 146: Wim Schoutens, Stochastic Processes and Orthogonal Polynomials, xiv, 163 pages, 2000.

Vol. 147: Jürgen Franke, Wolfgang Härdle, and Gerhard Stahl, Measuring Risk in Complex Stochastic Systems, xvi, 272 pages, 2000.

Vol. 148: S.E. Ahmed and Nancy Reid, Empirical Bayes and Likelihood Inference, x, 200 pages, 2000.

Vol. 149: D. Bosq, Linear Processes in Function Spaces: Theory and Applications, xv, 296 pages, 2000.

Vol. 150: Tadeusz Caliński and Sanpei Kageyama, Block Designs: A Randomization Approach, Volume I: Analysis, ix, 313 pages, 2000.

Vol. 151: Håkan Andersson and Tom Britton, Stochastic Epidemic Models and Their Statistical Analysis: ix, 152 pages, 2000.

4090220R00085

Made in the USA
San Bernardino, CA
29 August 2013